A FOOLPROOF WAY TO...

End
BACK
ATTACKS

Charles Templeton
Charles Godfrey, M.D.

KEY PORTER·BOOKS

Canadian Cataloguing in Publication Data

Templeton, Charles, 1915-
  End back attacks

Includes index.
ISBN 1-55013-321-7

1. Backache. I. Godfrey, Charles M., 1917-

RD771.B217T45   1991   617.5'64   C91-093314-6

Distributed in the United States by
Publishers Group West
4065 Hollis, Emeryville, CA 94608

Key Porter Books Limited
70 The Esplanade
Toronto, Ontario
Canada M5E 1R2

Typesetting: Computer Composition of Canada Inc.

Printed and bound in Canada

91 92 93 94 95 6 5 4 3 2 1

What one needs is a cast-iron back
with a hinge in it.
— Charles Dudley Warner

Contents

1

A Personal Word

AS VIVIDLY AS ANY EVENT IN MY LIFE, I [CHARLES Templeton] remember my first attack of acute back pain.

It happened in late September 1969. It was a Saturday. I had risen later than usual and was shaving, standing before the mirror in the bathroom. I smoked then and, having taken a last drag on a cigarette, half turned to toss it into the toilet bowl.

A stab of white-hot pain, followed immediately by excruciating agony across my entire lower back!

I howled and grasped the countertop, wondering what was happening, trying to keep from collapsing to the floor. My wife, in the kitchen, heard my cries and came running up the stairs, finding me immobilized and whimpering like a puppy. I glimpsed my face in the mirror; it was distorted and parchment white. A grayness began to close in.

"Quickly!" I said. "Get some ice. I'm going to faint."

She was back in a minute and applied a handful of ice cubes to the back of my neck. The grayness dissipated. I'm not sure how I got to the bed — crawling on my hands and knees, as best I recall it — but I do know that it took the better part of half an hour.

It was ten days before I was back on my feet, and another week before I could return to work.

THE BEGINNING OF A PATTERN

What caused the trauma? X-rays and a medical examination indicated that there was nothing organically wrong with my back. As best could be determined, the attack had resulted from an accumulation of intense and prolonged stress coupled with fatigue.

In the intervening twenty-two years I have suffered a number of such seizures (some of them comparably severe) as well as a variety of lesser episodes. Each time, the pattern became more evident — the onset followed an extended period of tension or fatigue and was triggered by a relatively minor incident. The lesser attacks tended to come less suddenly and were short- lived. They began as discomfort and increased in intensity over a period of hours, often overnight. Most of these followed overexertion during sports or unduly strenuous activity around the house. There was one common component: they all seemed related to periods of stress.

Since then I have learned through extensive reading and through conversations with other back-pain sufferers and with medical experts that, even though the specific circumstances of my afflictions and theirs may have differed considerably, some aspects of our common problems were alike and most of our symptoms were similar.

SEEKING THE CAUSE

Hoping to end this recurring problem, with all its inconvenience and pain, I decided two years ago to do an exhaustive examination of the available literature, to consult with specialists in the field and, if possible, to conquer my back problem. I had had enough of being deprived of certain activities and of nursing a nagging back. My objectives were threefold:

- to come to an understanding of the causes and effects of common back pain;
- to find ways to ease the pain and speed the recovery should I experience another acute attack; and,
- most important, to work out techniques that would enable me, if possible, to avoid future back attacks.

I soon discovered that the vast majority of back problems are simple and uncomplicated, that the reasons for their occurrence are not mysterious and that the onset of an attack can usually be forecast and guarded against.

I learned also that the great majority of back problems (more than 90 percent) do not require professional attention. They are, essentially, not much more complex than a sprained ankle.

VARIED OPINIONS

There is a considerable body of literature dealing with back problems. It ranges from scholarly treatises by medical specialists to a variety of pamphlets, many of the latter of limited or doubtful value. Some are faddist, fast-buck ripoffs. I found a wide divergence of opinion in some areas, much of it contradictory. The best sources provided informed data about the bone, musculature and nervous systems of the back and their interrelatedness.

There was much (far too much for the lay reader) about the various diseases and malformations that afflict the back but not enough specific counsel on how to deal with the pain during and immediately following an attack. Beyond that, most did not speak to the multiplicity of day-to-day problems faced by sufferers from back pain during the sometimes prolonged recovery period.

Despite their variety, they all seemed finally to make the same three fundamental points:

- that in fewer than 10 percent of cases, back trouble is related to disease or malformation of the spine;
- that, having suffered a back attack, you will fully recover within two to three months, *usually within a week to ten days*;
- that if, having recovered, you fail to follow a simple regimen of special exercises, you will suffer recurring back problems, each attack probably more severe than those preceding it.

FEW DETAILED INSTRUCTIONS

What I found lacking in most of these sources were specific suggestions on how to cope in daily life with a bad back. Most of the literature did not spell out in sufficient detail how to manage such mundane problems as:

- finding ways to rest comfortably in bed,
- taking a bath,
- bending over to pick up the morning newspaper or the baby in the playpen,
- straightening up after washing your hair, applying your makeup or brushing your teeth;
- sitting or standing for prolonged periods;
- maintaining bowel regularity;
- making love.

These and dozens of other simple, everyday activities can become complex problems in the initial recovery period. The victim needs inventive, practical help, and counsel on how to deal with the pain, the tension and the setbacks that are so often a part of the problem.

THE EMOTIONAL FACTOR

I learned early on that a large part of the affliction — perhaps the largest part — is related to the emotions. During the acute phase of an attack, fear is a constant companion, and even after you get back on your feet and return to normal life, it is never far away.

In the first hours and days of your recovery, you live with the fear of making a wrong move. You fret about the seriousness of your affliction. You brood about whether you dare do this or that, and whether this action or that might lead to a spasm or a setback, even put you back in bed.

Some sufferers from back pain become reluctant to leave the safety of home, not daring so much as to go to the store or even to visit the doctor's office.

DEALING WITH BACK PAIN

I decided to discuss my conclusions and the related medical questions with a long-time friend, Dr. Charles Godfrey, the man best equipped, in my opinion, to provide the relevant medical knowledge and the practical application of it. The result of our discussions was a decision to collaborate in the preparation of this book.

Our purpose is to present in straightforward layman's language the causes of common back pain, to explain why a so-called back attack happens and precisely what can be done about it. Our objective is to help make the recovery period less painful, less frightening and better understood and, more important, to enable the victim to end the cycle.

The various chapters of this book have been designed to remove that worst of fears, the fear of the unknown, and to explain exactly why your back hurts.

In these pages we discuss:

- the factors common to the onset of an acute "back attack,"
- the crucial first days of the recovery period,
- the immediate steps to take to reduce the pain,
- ways to counter and lessen anxiety,
- specific solutions to the problems of the bed-rest period,
- how to respond to your body's demands,
- how to get back on your feet again,
- how to manage your return to the workaday world, and,
- most importantly: *how to avoid a relapse by establishing in your subconscious mind what we call 'the automatic response system.'*

All the suggestions and techniques put forward in these pages are designed to make the pain more manageable, the dislocation of daily life less disruptive and the period of incapacitation shorter.

We will not deal here with the diseases and malformations of the spine, with such illnesses as arthritis, scoliosis, spondylitis, osteoporosis, spina bifida, herniated disc, etc. They cause a relatively small minority of back problems (fewer than ten percent) and should be treated by medical specialists. If you suffer from any abnormality or persistent back pain, the cause of which is not clear, discuss it with your family doctor.

Some of the recommendations will be familiar; they are the basics. Many of them will answer questions you have been asking and will help lessen the pain, the worry and the aggravation you have been enduring. Others may exorcise the demons of anxiety and fear that may have been bedeviling you.

What you do with them is up to you, but we offer this simple assurance — they work.

A PROFESSIONAL DIAGNOSIS

One imperative must be emphasized before proceeding. If you are suffering your first back attack or have never had a professional diagnosis of your problem, get one. The causes of some back problems — albeit a minority of them — are complex and varied, and self-diagnosis can be dangerous. Only a qualified medical specialist will know how to deal with them.

It is said of the layman who chooses to represent himself in court that he has "a fool for a lawyer and a fool for a client." It may just as aptly be said of the person who suffers a physical malady and diagnoses his own problem that he has "a fool for a doctor and a fool for a patient."

But if you have been examined by a competent professional and are suffering no new symptoms, get ready to slough off most of the fear, much of the pain and a lot of the inconvenience that can beset the person who is afflicted with what is commonly described as "a bad back."

2

Dealing with an Acute Attack

THERE IS A SHARP, EXCRUCIATING PAIN IN YOUR back, like the sudden thrust of a knife.

It has struck without warning or perhaps after signaling its onset with dull discomfort over a period of hours. However it may have originated, the acute phase has come, and you are bent over in agony or immobilized on your bed.

What to do?

If this is your first experience with major back pain, you should, of course, contact your family doctor. If, however, the pain in your back is no new thing, if you are one of those millions of men and women who have a recurring back problem, certain measures must be taken.

There are two immediate imperatives: to control the pain and to maintain control of your emotions.

DEALING WITH AN ACUTE ATTACK

An acute back attack can cause agony, making even the strongest of us cry out and fall to the floor in a faint. In some cases, the victim may be temporarily incapacitated.

Fortunately, the onset is not usually that dramatic.

Acute back pain varies with the individual. It may begin with little more than a slight twinge and intensify overnight to pain that will leave you bedridden for days. It may be the result of attempting to lift too heavy a load, the collision of bodies on the field of sports, working too long in the garden. It may be caused by an extended period of tension or by as simple a thing as bending over to pick up the morning paper, suddenly correcting a loss of balance, exposure to a cold draft, even a vigorous sneeze.

And the pain can manifest itself in a variety of areas: in the low back, at mid-back, in the buttocks, in the legs, in a shoulder or in the neck.

However the onset begins and whatever the characteristics of the attack, the result is often severe pain. And that pain must be dealt with as expeditiously as possible.

Commonly, in an acute attack, the muscles of the back have been subjected to more stress than they can handle and have suffered injury. Not infrequently, some of the muscle fibres tear. There may be internal bleeding and, as a consequence, local swelling.

But the most severe pain in an acute attack usually comes from a secondary source: spasm in the surrounding muscles as the body attempts to minimize damage in the affected area, and it is imperative that this spasm be eased as soon as possible; the longer the muscles remain locked in spasm, the more irritated they become, which can itself prolong the seizure.

MUSCLE SPASM

You are probably familiar with muscle spasm, having experienced it in the form of a cramp in the calf of your leg. Such cramping often happens in bed at night. The muscles contract and seize, usually pulling the ball of the foot downward. The pain is intense. How is it relieved? Typically, by putting an increasing amount of your weight on the foot and slowly stretching the muscles until the contraction eases. Sometimes the seized muscles can be relaxed with vigorous massage, by applying heat or by "walking it off."

Recalling such an experience will help you to understand what happens when the muscles of your back go into spasm. Just as muscle spasm produces severe pain in the calf of your leg, a similar muscular contraction can cause severe pain in the muscles of your back.

Usually, you can ease the spasm in your calf within minutes. And, when you do, the pain diminishes almost immediately. Indeed, apart from a slight soreness, it may be gone entirely within a few minutes.

This same sequence can take place in your back, and that is why it is important to know what is causing your pain and what needs to be done to relieve it. We'll get to that in a moment.

Part of the problem of dealing with muscle spasm in the back is that you may find yourself immobilized by fear. You think to yourself: such a severe pain *must* be dangerous. You may panic, fearing that, if you so much as *move*, the pain will get worse. Intensifying this fear is the primal concern we feel about injuries to the back.

You may be immobilized also by the reaction of your autonomic nervous system. The autonomic nervous system is not controlled by the brain. It reacts automatically; in this case immobilizing the muscles surrounding the injury by going into spasm. It is the body's mechanism for limiting the damage.

It is important to be aware of the nature of this involuntary "protective" intervention. You did not initiate the spasm and you cannot easily end it. It is an instance of the body overcompensating. You can no more *will* your seized back muscles to relax than you could *will* your cramped calf muscles to release.

Unfortunately, with back spasm there is no comparably simple action to be taken to relieve the cramp as there is in the case of the seized muscle in your calf; it is a matter of making do as best you can in the circumstances. What you should try to do is get into a position that will enable you to stretch the back muscles and thus return them to normal.

Your best option may be to sit on the floor or on a chair and hug your knees to your chest. If you can, get onto a bed. Lie on your back or on your side, whichever is more convenient or more comfortable.

STRETCHING THE MUSCLES

The goal now is *gently but firmly to stretch the contracted muscles until they release and return to normal.* The pain may be intense, but you must persevere. Hang tough, and you may soon feel a dramatic easing of the pain.

The bad news is, of course, that the pain might not pass. There are no guarantees, but the strong likelihood is that it will ease.

You should be aware that, if the pain does ease, there still remains the possibility of intermittent spasms. Get into bed as expeditiously as possible and concentrate on relaxing. If you can, get into the fetal position. And talk to yourself. Remind yourself that what is happening will surely pass. Remember, too, that it poses no threat to your health. As the familiar phrase goes: "It may hurt you but it won't harm you."

You may wish to sit in a low chair and lean as far forward as you can; your hands clutching your ankles, your head low, your chin tucked in. Assume this position slowly but firmly.

An acquaintance responds to his back going into spasm by lying on the floor and putting his feet flat against the wall, his buttocks as close to the wall as is feasible. Sounds awkward, but he swears it is unfailingly effective. Another friend lies on the floor and tries to rest the calves of his legs on a chair or coffee table, getting his buttocks as close as possible. A woman, interviewed on television, said that she squats in a corner, held secure by the intersecting walls, and bends the trunk of her body as far forward as she can. She didn't say how she gets out of the corner once the pain has eased and how she avoids cramps in her thighs, but, if it works, who is to tell her nay.

The fact is there there are no inflexible rules, there is no universal panacea. But knowing what you need to accomplish may enable you to find a solution that is effective for you.

FIGHTING FEAR

As mentioned earlier, a large part of the problem during an acute back attack is fear. The fear is understandable, but you must try to contain it. Not to do so will make the situation worse. Often, tension is a major cause of a back attack, and fear creates and intensifies tension. You must try to counter it.

Have a "Dutch uncle" talk with yourself — aloud, if it helps. Remind yourself forcefully that, despite the severity of the pain, you are in no mortal danger. Difficult as it may be to do, remind yourself that what is happening will soon pass, and that it is in your power to help end it by mastering your fear.

Easier said than done, but essential.

STAYING PUT
The crisis has passed and you are now in bed. Stay there. Get up as little as possible — not at all, if you can manage it.

Some years ago, having suffered a very painful attack, the victim telephoned his doctor, an old friend, seeking advice. The doctor was too busy to come to the telephone, but called back after a few minutes.

"I'm told your back's acting up," he said.

The patient recited an extended litany of symptoms and woes and ended by asking his friend what he should do.

The doctor responded by asking, "Where are you calling from?"

"My bed."

"Stay there," he said brusquely. "Take the maximum doses of a coated aspirin and come see me when you're back on your feet."

That was the end of the conversation. The victim was offended by his old friend's matter-of-factness. It was only as three days passed and he was able to get up and about again that he realized he had been given the best advice possible.

Bed rest.

It is by long odds the most effective "treatment" following an acute attack. Analgesics, heat and cold, muscle relaxants, manipulation, massage, ointments, hot showers, whirlpool baths, vibrators — the list goes on and on — may be helpful, but they are all supplementary. First and foremost, the injured muscles need time to heal. And total inactivity — for *at least* the first day or two — is essential to the achievement of that purpose.

PROFESSIONAL COUNSEL

If you have just suffered your first back attack or find yourself with symptoms unlike any you have previously experienced, it is imperative that, before doing anything else, you seek professional advice.

Do not try to be your own doctor or to make your own diagnosis. Nor should you let other amateurs counsel you. No matter how much you may have read on the subject, and despite any suggestions from well-meaning but uninformed friends, the ailments to which the human back is subject are many and complex, and the symptoms can be misleading. You need the advice of a trained specialist.

So, first, talk to your family doctor.

If your problem is a straightforward one, an obvious case of common back sprain, a doctor's examination will reveal this and, if nothing else, will free your mind of the unreasonable fears that victims of back pain are subject to. If your doctor does not feel equipped to deal with your problem, he or she will refer you to a specialist, which will at least keep you from turning to quacks, of which there are not a few.

Herewith, a few comments on the various sources of diagnosis and treatment.

Your family doctor

In seeking help for your back problem, you should consult first with your family doctor.

There are many reasons for doing so. Not least, your doctor will know your medical history, which could be relevant. He or she will also know something of your personality and your idiosyncracies; this can be useful, particularly because back trouble is so often related to the personality of the victim and to the emotions.

Medical doctors do two things: they diagnose and they treat. Their training and practice equip them to do this. That training continues in the daily practice of medicine: in the treatment of patients suffering various illnesses and exhibiting (or describing) an infinite variety of symptoms.

In general, no one is better equipped initially to treat or counsel you about your back than a good general practitioner.

That is the ideal; the reality may differ. There are doctors and there are doctors. Most are competent and conscientious, but doctors are human beings and as such are subject to bias, preoccupation, carelessness and errors in judgment.

One first-rate general practitioner had "a blind eye and a deaf ear" when it came to problems of the back. Apart from those illnesses of the spine that could be diagnosed as diseases or malformations, he regarded back pain as more nuisance than illness, characterized all chiropractors as "spine thumpers" and dismissed most complaints about back pain with the advice: "Soak in a hot Epsom-salts bath and take it easy for a day or two. You're not as young as you used to be."

As a further example of how even highly trained physicians can err, an eminent Canadian psychiatrist commonly dismisses back pain with the comment, "The biggest reason for back pain is to get a sick-leave ticket from the Workers' Compensation office."

These professionals are the exception, however, and the evidence would suggest that they are among a diminishing minority. An increasing number of general practitioners now accept the validity of manipulation and other hands-on techniques as viable alternatives and, if they don't themselves offer extensive treatment, frequently make referrals to osteopaths, physiotherapists, chiropractors or other back specialists.

Those MDs who do provide treatment usually — as their discipline prescribes — insist on making a diagnosis before beginning it. In this they often differ from non-medical manipulators, too many of whom will proceed to treatment after only a superficial examination.

Chiropractors

Chiropractors are and have long been the focus of controversy in the treatment of illness. As mentioned above, there are medical doctors who damn them indiscriminately, even as there are others who not infrequently refer patients to them. As well, there are patients who, having been helped by chiropractors, hail them as wonder-workers, and others who dismiss them as quacks.

Chiropractic was founded by a Canadian-born American, Daniel Palmer, just before the turn of the century and, after a long battle to establish its credibility, has flourished increasingly. In the early years, many chiropractors claimed that the manipulation of the spine provided a comprehensive system for the treatment of virtually all illnesses. There has been a considerable retrenching related to this claim and a subsequent addition of a number of more or less exotic services. They include massage, acupuncture, herbal remedies, ultrasound, colonic irrigation, iridology, hydrotherapy, reflexology, intestinal manipulation, therapeutic touch, aromatherapy and aesthetics.

As well, patients commonly have pressed on them literature stressing vegetarianism and other holistic health regimens.

For all this, there are many highly competent and skillful chiropractors, men and women who diligently and intelligently seek to provide effective treatment for a variety of ills — and, in many cases, do. But chiropractic is not the optimum treatment for many conditions, and the patient who does not see significant improvement after two weeks of treatment would be well advised to seek a second opinion elsewhere.

If there is one fault common to chiropractic treatment it is the tendency of the practitioner to insist on partial or whole-body X-rays before proceeding to treatment. The result can be excessive and often unnecessary radiation.

Can a skilled chiropractor help you with certain back problems? The answer is an unequivocal yes. However, a minority of them seem to have as a principal concern the moving of patients in and out of the multiple treatment rooms as expeditiously as possible. Do some chiropractors confuse you with doubletalk, cajole you into routine visits when the need has passed and seek to sell you a variety of products and services of borderline value? Again, the answer is yes.

Osteopaths

If your symptoms indicate a need for manipulation of the spine or specialized treatment of the the nerves and muscles of the back, legs, neck and shoulders, your GP will be more likely to refer you to an osteopath than to a chiropractor.

One reason that osteopaths are the preferred referral may well be that the educational prerequisites for their licensing are similar to those required for a medical degree, the only major difference being that the osteopath gets his or her training at a school of osteopathy rather than at a traditional medical school.

Osteopaths, while they specialize in manipulative therapy, are licensed to treat a variety of other seemingly unrelated illnesses such as high blood pressure and diabetes. In Canada, they practice under the same laws as chiropractors and are not permitted to prescribe drugs. In the United States, they are fully qualified medically, and some, with additional training, perform surgery.

Although both the chiropractor and the osteopath specialize in manipulation of the spine, the osteopath tends to put more emphasis on leverage in making adjustments and will more likely employ specialized massage, manual traction and a repetitive stretching of the ligaments around a joint in order to correct a misalignment or to return an area to full mobility. The emphasis tends to be on freeing and easing rather than on thrusting or applying force.

There can be little doubt that manipulation therapy can be useful in treating a bad back — whether performed by a skilled MD, a chiropractor, an osteopath or a physical therapist. Pain can be relieved in many, if not in most cases, whether it involves a release from muscle spasm, facet-joint misalignment, chronic muscular tension or other ills related to the spine.

Incidentally, if you wish to see a local osteopath or chiropractor, no referral by an MD is necessary. You simply call for an appointment. Nevertheless, it would be wise to check in advance with your doctor and get his or her advice. The doctor may (or may not) wish to refer you or to forward medical information to the practitioner of your choice, and such data might be useful in your treatment.

Generally, an osteopath's patients tend to be either dismissive or enthusiastic advocates of their practitioner's skills. Some are almost zealots.

Acupuncture

Even though it is the oldest form of medical treatment known to man, you will find no unanimity of opinion in the health community on the effectiveness of acupuncture as a treatment for back problems.

There is reference to the system in the earliest recorded treatise on medicine, one purportedly written by the Yellow Emperor, Huang Ti, around 2600 B.C.

Western medicine was introduced to the system some two hundred years ago and tended to dismiss it as conceptually interesting but medically unsound. This view has altered significantly in recent years, and many in orthodox medical circles have come to accept the validity of the method in treating certain illnesses — even while they are uncertain as to how it works.

There is now considerable agreement that acupuncture is a legitimate means of treatment in certain circumstances, primarily for the relief of pain and as an anesthetic during treatment for various ills. More recently it has been approved in the United States for the management of chronic pain, neuralgia and arthritis. In some cases the relief seems to be long-term, even permanent. In other cases, the pain continues unabated or eases briefly and returns after a few hours or days.

Acupuncture is based on the Taoist philosophy that good health depends on the state of a life-force energy (T'chi) throughout the organs of the body. It is believed that physical, and even mental, health depend on a harmonious balance between *yin* and *yang* — *yin* being negative, cold, passive, dark, hidden, solid and female; *yang* being positive, warm, active, light, open, hollow and male. (How's that for an example of early sexism!)

The goal of the practitioner is to correct any imbalance between these opposite forces (which permit discord and disease) and to allow the body's natural healing mechanisms to be dominant.

The ancient Chinese worked out on the body a series of what are called "points." Each point (there are about eight hundred) represents a specific organ or part of the body. These points have been organized along an interconnected system of fourteen main lines, or "meridians," that run from head to foot on both sides of the body.

The goal of acupuncture is to identify the imbalance in *yin* and *yang* energy that, it is believed, is causing the illness, and by inserting very fine needles into certain points and vibrating or twirling them, to stimulate (or retard) the flow of energy until the imbalance has been corrected. The body then heals itself.

Acupuncture undoubtedly has some effectiveness, although it appears to work better on some types of pain and on certain types of individuals. Indeed, the best results seem to be achieved with what might be described as a particular personality type.

Those determined to dismiss the treatment as purely psychological should note that specific results have been achieved with acupuncture on animals as well as humans.

It is anything but clear why acupuncture works. It is posited that, when chronic "pain patterns" have set in, the cycle may be broken by acupuncture, perhaps by a relaxing of the nervous system or by a blocking of certain "pain pathways," perhaps even by releasing the body's own painkilling hormones, the endorphins and encephalins.

Western medicine is just beginning to use acupuncture as a means for treating pain. If your particular affliction is longstanding and has not responded to more conventional methods, you may wish to try it. There are numerous testimonials as to its effectiveness in treating certain ailments.

Hypnotherapy

Hypnosis does not serve as a cure for a serious back condition but has been shown to be useful as a means for controlling chronic back pain by affecting the perception of pain and by reducing tension.

It is also employed to help the patient gain access to subconscious functions in the brain and thus to affect the operation of the body's autonomic system, the operative mechanism engendering muscle spasm.

Hypnotism (the word derives from the Greek for "putting to sleep") was first known as "Animal Magnetism and Mesmerism" (after the German physician Franz Anton Mesmer, who experimented in the treatment of psychosomatic illnesses in the late eighteenth century). It came into vogue in the late nineteenth and early twentieth centuries but was viewed by most as little more than a vaudeville trick until taken seriously by, among others, a group of French medical researchers seeking to deal effectively with hysteria and to probe the subconscious. It was used for a time by Sigmund Freud in psychoanalysis and is still widely employed as a technique by psychotherapists to induce relaxation or to help sufferers from amnesia to recall traumatic events.

Patients are led by the therapist into a trance state superficially resembling sleep, during which attempts are made to examine thoughts, images and perceptions; to produce feelings of relaxation, equanimity and calmness; to recall traumatic events; to alter unpleasant memories and, later, to refashion patients' perception of themselves, their pain and their reactions to it.

Hypnotherapy can be a useful if limited treatment for some individuals with back problems, mostly in the reduction of tension, the easing of chronic pain and the control of muscular spasm. Studies have shown that back-pain sufferers can be, and have been, helped by it but the numbers are not large and the individuals benefiting tend to be of a certain personality type.

Will it work for you? It is impossible to say; much of the effectiveness of the treatment depends on the patient and on the skill of the hypnotherapist. Will it do harm? Apparently not. Indeed, if nothing else, it may help the individual to relax and to learn self-hypnosis, a useful tool in relieving tension.

There are other treatments, of course — more, in fact, than can be dealt with here, many of them obscure. A few make plausible claims and have their advocates; others are little more than quackery.

3

Managing the Pain

UNLESS YOU ARE A MASOCHIST OR INTENT ON demonstrating your Spartan qualities, there is no point in suffering needless back pain. And there *are* things you can do to ease it.

Pain is not the enemy; it is an ally. It is not the problem; it is a symptom. It is an alarm-bell, a danger signal, a warning. It says: "Pay attention; something's wrong. Do something about it."

A friend was in automobile accident on a country road and had no option but to walk some distance to find help. In shock and, as a consequence, feeling no pain, he did not realize that he had fractured an ankle and, in the long walk to find help, aggravated the injury. Normally, the pain produced each time he put his weight on the ankle would have served to protect him against the damage.

To suffer back pain and disregard it is to be a fool. Heed the signal; it will help you to avoid more serious problems.

Fear is an emotion. And as is true of most intense emotions, it can affect both the body and the psyche. It is one of the body's protective mechanisms, its purpose being to preserve you from danger.

Much of the distress in a painful situation is not the pain but the fear of more pain. Such is surely true of back pain. Back pain ranges from the agony of muscles ruptured or in spasm, to pressures on a nerve, to facet-joint misalignment, to residual soreness. Viewed objectively, the day-to-day pain of the recovery period is not intense. Most of the time it is a localized soreness — unpleasant but bearable.

But after an acute back attack, the compounding factor is that fear is in bed with you. The agony of the initial seizure is fresh in your memory. And there are, inevitably, brief episodes in which, making a wrong move, you induce a jab of sharp pain. If this aftermath pain were the only problem, we could handle it without much concern . The reason for the overconcern is that we live with *the overriding fear that the original pain is about to return*.

In such circumstances each of us reacts differently:

- Some freeze. Tense as a spring, fearful as a paranoid, they lie rigid, immobilized, steeling themselves against the next onset.
- Some dwell on the problem. They stay in bed longer than necessary, fretting about their condition, postponing getting up and generally feeling sorry for themselves.
- Some try to disregard the affliction. "The office can't run without me." "The baby has to be fed." "Meals have to be made." "I'm not going to let a sore back keep *me* in bed."

- Some use good sense. They try to look at the problem with objectivity ("It sure isn't funny but it's not fatal"). They do what can be done to handle the pain. And they use the time in bed as an opportunity: to do some planning, to gain a perspective on their life, to catch up on their reading, to write some overdue letters.

USE THE HELP THAT IS AVAILABLE

It is interesting to note that, after incurring most injuries, we usually take immediate steps to treat them. Sprain an ankle and we immobilize it. Sustain a cut and we hasten to the medicine cabinet for something to sterilize the wound and to stop the bleeding. Burn a finger and we apply a cream or ointment. Break a tooth and we dash to the dentist.

But, with an attack of back pain, too many do little more than groan, curse their luck, take a couple of aspirins and grimly soldier on, thus delaying and possibly complicating the recovery. Such behavior may seem courageous, but it is foolish. It is unwise to disregard pain of any kind. If the symptom is familiar and you know its pattern, well and good — treat it. But if what you are suffering is something new and it is severe enough to disturb or dominate your day, check into it.

There are, of course, those who overreact, who flee to their bed for the most trivial reasons, who call their doctor daily, who grimace at every twinge, who walk to the bathroom as though on thin ice and become a quivering mass of anticipatory tension. I think of them as "back-pain layabouts," Their number is legion.

Try to be neither cavalier nor craven.

THE FIVE WORST KINDS OF PAIN

There are learned studies on the phenomenon of pain and its relative severity. Some years ago an article in a medical journal sought to describe the five worst kinds of commonly endured pain. The clinician listed them — in no particular order — as the passing of a kidney stone, a difficult childbirth, infection of the inner ear, certain types of cancer and acute back pain.

Not to suggest that common back pain is comparable to a session on the medieval rack; it isn't. But neither is it a summer picnic in the park.

The point we are seeking to make is this: in the initial stage of an acute attack, there are a number of things you can *do* to ease the pain and repair the damage, and it is foolish to neglect or disdain them.

THE PAINKILLERS

The first thing to be done after an acute attack is to take action to alleviate the pain.

One of the universally available painkillers should be your first recourse, not simply because enduring needless pain is pointless but because the injured muscles and nerves of your back are in the process of becoming inflamed, swelling and possibly beginning a chain-reaction of muscle spasm.

The immediate question is, of course, which of the much-touted analgesics you should use. The answer is not necessarily the clichéd "Take two aspirins and call me in the morning," nor is it to dose yourself indiscriminately with one of the dozens of painkillers trumpeted on the television screen as being superior to and more powerful than their rivals.

Each maker of a universally available painkiller claims its own to be different from and better than the competition, and laymen, confused by the plethora of conflicting claims, come to the conclusion that the clamor is no more than promotional hype and that the various products are essentially the same.

Not so. There are significant differences related to effectiveness and safety that determine which palliative you should take for your back pain.

Acetylsalicylic acid

The best-known and most frequently used of the common pain-relievers is ASA (acetylsalicylic acid). It is extracted from the bark of the white willow, and its extraordinary ability to alleviate pain and reduce fever and inflammation has been recognized for centuries.

ASA is best known the world over by the name "Aspirin," the famous Bayer trademark. The other well-known brands (Anacin, Bufferin, Excedrin, etc.) claim to be different and superior (and, in some ways, may be) but all contain ASA as their principal ingredient. Some add codeine in sufficiently small amounts to enable them to remain available as nonprescription drugs. Other varieties include some form of coating or chemical "buffer" to counter potential acidic irritation in the stomach. Others add caffeine as a stimulant, but, in each case, the effective ingredient is the ASA.

If you are not subject to stomach irritation on taking ASA, you may wish to try a product called Robaxisal. It is a powerful nonprescription analgesic and muscle relaxant and, if not on the shelves, is often available simply by asking for it at the pharmacist's counter. A prescription may be required in the USA. In addition to the usual amount of ASA, it contains 8 mg of codeine phosphate and 400 mg of methocarbamol, a muscle-relaxant.

One of the principal causes of back pain when muscle damage has occurred is the inflammation that follows it. In simple terms, inflammation is the immediate reaction of your body to an injury. Its purpose is to help the injured tissue repair itself. In doing so, the body's mechanisms produce heat, redness, swelling and pain.

The point to be borne in mind in taking a pain-reliever is this: if you need it, *take it!* Don't stew about it. And take it in sufficient dosages to get the benefit from it. Don't take the least amount possible; analgesics are most useful when taken as directed since their effectiveness is much greater when blood levels of the ingredients are maintained.

Most men and women can take ASA in the prescribed amounts — two 325 mg tablets every four hours as needed. Do not exceed twelve tablets daily. Check the label. This dosage will not only reduce your pain, but will also act to reduce the inflammation at the site of the injury where, as a result of the damage to the muscles or ligaments, localized bleeding may have occurred.

Drink a large glass of water with each dosage and, as with all drugs, *do not deviate from the dosages listed on the label and stop using it if you notice any adverse reaction.*

However, for all its effectiveness as an analgesic and as a powerful anti-inflammatory agent, ASA can pose problems for a minority of users — upset stomach, constipation, even gastric bleeding — and can interfere with the normal coagulation of the blood. If you notice any complications or side-effects of consequence, stop taking it.

The acetaminophens

The second major group of pain-relievers, the acetaminophens, were first prescribed late in the nineteenth century and are cheap and effective analgesics.

They are also useful in controlling fever. Marketed under such brand names as Tylenol, Exodol and Atasol, they have the virtue of not irritating the stomach. Unfortunately, they do not have anti-inflammatory properties, important in palliating muscle damage and some other causes of back pain. They, too, are available with codeine and caffeine added.

Both ASA and the acetaminophens are available in "extra-strength" forms. This means merely that they contain more than the usual amounts of ASA. You can check their relative strengths by comparing labels. As with ASA, do not exceed the recommended dosages on the label.

The ibuprofens

More recently, a new type of analgesic has appeared on the market: NSAIDs (nonsteroid anti-inflamatory drugs), best-known as the ibuprofens.

Developed originally to combat arthritic pain, they are an effective pain-reliever and, notably, are useful in reducing inflammation. The best-known brands are Motrin, Nuprin and Actiprofen. Unfortunately, the ibuprofens also have their drawbacks: they sometimes produce stomach problems, even gastric hemorrhage, and can cause kidney and liver dysfunction in the elderly. They may also induce allergic symptoms, especially in people who react adversely to ASA.

It must be emphasized that none of the analgesics described above will entirely relieve most acute back pain or the severe pain of muscle spasm. But they can help and should be used as needed.

ADVERSE REACTIONS

If you are on other medications or have a history of heart, circulatory, kidney or stomach problems, or if you experience dizziness or other significant side-effects after taking the medications listed above, check with your doctor, or talk to your pharmacist. If you have any reason for doubt or are suffering *any* adverse reaction of consequence, stop taking the medication immediately.

If this is your first experience with back pain (or if you are an old-hand but experiencing unfamiliar symptoms), don't doctor yourself. Most back pain is uncomplicated and will, with bed rest and controlled activity, generally heal itself, but it can be complex and serious, and if you are in any doubt as to its cause, get professional attention.

PUTTING THE PAIN ON ICE

During the first twenty-four hours you may find it helpful to apply cold to the affected area. Cold will do two things: it will reduce the pain somewhat by desensitizing the peripheral nerves in the area and it will counter and help contain the swelling.

Your immediate inclination may be to apply heat — and there are some who advocate this — but heat can increase the swelling and the stiffness because of increased surface circulation, and that you don't need at this stage. If, however, you find the application of a heating-pad or a hot-water bottle soothing, by all means use it; it will do no harm.

Cold is not as comfortable or soothing as heat — which is one of the reasons it is described as a counterirritant — but this characteristic can make it an effective treatment during the first forty-eight hours. No one is quite certain why a counterirritant is effective. It is thought that the acute sensation it produces may block the transmission of the pain signal to the brain or that applying it may cause the brain to release endorphins, the body's powerful anesthetic, into the bloodstream.

Whatever the reason, cold can be helpful in the early hours — not least because it constricts the capillaries (the smallest blood-carrying vessels) and can thus reduce internal bleeding. As well, it has a numbing effect, and with this diminution of the pain, you may find it possible — if you are suffering muscle spasm — to begin to stretch the contracted muscles in the area (cautiously, at first), thus easing that problem.

Applying ice

It is no easy thing to apply cold to yourself — indeed, you may find that you are not so much as able to get out of bed even to do the preparation — so get help if you can.

If you own an icepack, half-fill it with crushed ice and apply it to the sore area. If you don't have an icepack, one can be fashioned by crushing some ice and placing it in a plastic freezer bag.

An unorthodox but effective option is a bag of frozen peas fresh from the freezer. Drop the bag on the counter-top a time or two to free the individual peas. Incidentally, it isn't an extravagance; you can return it to the freezer and use it again and again — although not to eat, of course.

Insulate the icepack by wrapping it in a small towel so that it won't cause frostbite. Don't overwrap it; it will then do little good. Apply it to the affected area of your back for twenty minutes, but no longer.

A more effective method is to apply the ice directly to the skin. A spouse or friend should take a paper cup (or better, a styrofoam cup), fill it with cold water and place it in the freezer compartment of the refrigerator.

When it is frozen solid, tear away the open-end half of the cup, exposing some of the ice but leaving the bottom of the cup as an insulator for the fingers. It may help to wrap a couple of facial tissues around the covered portion to improve the insulation.

Ideally, the patient should lie face down on the bed. You may find it useful to place a small pillow under the

stomach to avoid arching the back, and you should certainly remove the pillow from beneath your head. Even
with the pillow supporting your midriff, the position may
be too painful. If it intensifies the pain, stop — it could
indicate that the problem is not simply muscular.

Alternatively, try lying on your side in the fetal position
with your knees drawn up, or with one knee drawn up,
permitting you to half-turn onto your stomach.

If the pain is on both sides of the spine, massage each
separately, rotating the ice in a slow circular motion. It is
not necessary or wise to apply pressure. The application
of the ice is not a form of massage but is an attempt to
desensitize the area and to contain the inflammation.

The person applying the ice should warn you before
making each contact. Unless you anticipate the shock,
your reaction to the cold could cause you to flinch or pull
away, which could initiate a spasm.

The ice should not be applied directly to the spine. It
won't do any harm but neither will it do any good, and the
bumpy ride can be painful.

Do not exceed seven minutes of constant application
on either side — there is the possibility of frostbite. A
maximum time of ten to twelve minutes to do both sides
is enough.

And don't trust your mental clock; time it.

The melting ice can be messy, so position a bath towel
to absorb the water as it runs down your back toward the
bedsheets.

Going it alone

Applying the ice is a tricky business to do yourself. The
trip to the kitchen, the preparation of the ice and the
application of it to your own back are forbiddingly difficult, if not impossible, procedures during the early hours

of a back attack — and that is when the ice is most beneficial.

If, nevertheless, you decide to proceed, position the icepack with one hand behind your back while lying on one side and then the other. If you intend to apply the ice directly, remember to protect your fingers from the cold and to absorb the runoff or you will be uncomfortable on soggy sheets after the treatment.

And remember to keep careful account of the time.

APPLYING HEAT

There is some difference of opinion among professionals as to whether heat is useful in the treatment of back pain — indeed, there is no unanimity on the benefits of cold — but neither can do any harm, and many advocate their use. We have found heat beneficial.

It would seem unwise to use heat during the first forty-eight hours when your immediate objectives are to contain the inflammation and the swelling.

The principal benefit of heat would seem to be that it helps relax the muscles (and you), and this is certainly useful in treating muscle spasm. It is probable that the benefit derives from the increased circulation of blood in the afflicted area — the heat stimulating the blood flow, which then carries away the wastes resulting from any internal bleeding or swelling that may have taken place at the site.

Some medical doctors and chiropractors insist that a heating-pad is not a particularly effective means of treatment, and suggest that, if heat is used, it should be *moist* heat. (One cannot but wonder why moist heat, inasmuch as the moisture does not penetrate the skin.) Nevertheless, if such is your doctor's counsel, there is no reason not to follow it. Moist or not, heat should not be applied for more than thirty minutes.

If you have a heating-pad, try it. It *is* relaxing. As a concession to the advocates of moist heat, you might experiment by placing a layer of plastic wrap against the skin, with a towel between it and the heating-pad. It certainly does produce moisture in the form of perspiration.

There can be no doubt, however, about one form of moist heat: immersion in a warm tub or, better, the direct flow of warm water onto the affected area while in the shower (see Chapter 9). Not only is it a balm for your sore back, it will do your sagging spirits a world of good.

MASSAGE

Massage is a dicey activity in the early hours and days of a back attack. On the other hand, it can have a soothing effect if the person applying it is sensitive to your heightened apprehension and to the sometimes unpredictability of muscle spasm.

Muscle spasm is involuntary, that is, it is not within your control, and is a reflex action in the muscles surrounding the injury. Its purpose is to immobilize and protect the area from further damage. Unfortunately, this reaction can be triggered by massage and this will, in itself, enforce an end to the session.

However, there is a kind of nonspecific muscle tension in the back, commonly produced by apprehension, that can be reduced by firm but careful massage. A skillful and caring partner can be exceedingly helpful during the recovery period, and if you have this kind of help available, you may wish to purchase a book on the subject and thus increase the benefits. Larger book stores and stores that specialize in serving victims of back pain probably carry such how-tos.

If liniment or ointment is being applied while you stand or have turned onto your stomach, take particular care. If an excess of zeal is shown, the result could be painful. Although the person performing the massage is only trying to help, too much pressure can produce a short-lived but painful spasm.

Self-massage

Of the various methods for relaxing the muscles of the back, you may find self-massage by far the most useful. We recommend it unreservedly from the acute phase through the recovery period, when there is residual stiffness, soreness or the odd twinge of pain in the affected area.

It is particularly useful first thing in the morning, when your muscles are stiff from sleep, or when you have been sitting or standing in one position for an extended time. During bad times, use it as often as a dozen or more times a day. With time, it will become an almost automatic response to stiffness or pain in the area.

Best of all, it is easy to do and can be done virtually anywhere.

While standing, place the palms of your hands on the small of the back, the thumbs somewhere near the top of the hip bones where they can provide a kind of anchor and some leverage. Massage the area on each side of the spine, with emphasis on the up-stroke of the fingers. Pay particular attention to the pain areas.

Because you are the masseur/masseuse, you can control the pressure, using as much or as little as you find helpful.

Once you have the hang of it, experiment with various strokes and varying amounts of pressure. Move from area to area, kneading as strongly as feels appropriate. Try using the heel of your hands on the back, or along the bottom of the ribcage, or around each side and toward the front.

Begin during the period of bed rest. Lie on your side and massage the affected area. Your body will tell you how much pressure to use. You may find it occasionally painful early on; you will also find it beneficial.

Once you are out of bed, get in the habit of massaging the vulnerable area regularly. A minute or so is sufficient, whenever you feel the need.

You need not apply your fingers directly to the skin; you can work through your clothing. And the technique can as readily be used while sitting. Simply lean slightly forward and begin. Not only is massage beneficial in easing the tension in the muscles, it increases the blood flow in the area.

As a way to relax tight or fatigued muscles and ease soreness — especially in a touch-and-go situation when you can't get off your feet — nothing is more immediately effective. Self-massage can ease or ward off any number of minor attacks.

Acquire the habit.

SALVES, LINIMENTS AND OINTMENTS
You may find it useful to use ointments or liniments from time to time for the benefits of so-called deep heat. There is a large variety available, ranging from the old-fashioned "horse liniment" to highly aromatic ointments and even pharmacological salves that contain ASA.

The "heat" produced by these salves and liniments won't penetrate the sore muscles, of course — the effect is purely peripheral — but some of them do produce a feeling of permeating heat, burning or tingling, and it is entirely possible that the sensation acts as a counterirritant, helping to block the pain signals from the injured muscles.

As with any form of treatment in seeking to relieve the tension and discomfort related to back pain, if it helps, use it.

4

Understanding the Problem

YOU ARE IN BED AS THE RESULT OF A SEVERE back attack.

The seizure may have come with the suddenness of a bolt of lightning or with a slight soreness that intensified with the passage of the hours. However it began — as the result of an accident, overdoing it on the tennis court, careless lifting on the job, reaching for the top shelf in the kitchen or lifting the baby out of the playpen — whether it is the recurrence of a longstanding problem or your first back attack, you are in bed, in considerable pain, and it is clear you are going to have to stay put — at the very least, for a few days.

As you begin your sojourn in bed, it is important to understand something of the nature and dimensions of your problem.

FACING THE REALITY

An acute back attack is a serious problem, but it is not life-threatening. You have not done yourself permanent injury. In all likelihood, you will be back to normal in a few days, or at most a few weeks. Nevertheless, it is an illness of consequence and must be treated as such. Try to dismiss it with macho stoicism as something to be conquered by sheer will-power and you will only worsen the predicament. One man, a strong-willed, self-assertive fellow, smitten with a back attack, rejected bed rest as weakness and thus exacerbated his problem and doubled the recovery period.

But he is the exception. The opposite reaction is more likely.

Many men and women, having endured the agonizing pain of an acute back attack, develop an abnormal fear of a recurrence. More often than not it is because they misunderstand the nature of their affliction and convince themselves — often despite the reassurances of their doctors — that they have done themselves major, perhaps permanent harm.

And they are full of misinformation:
- They believe the spine is a fragile thing — it is not.
- They believe they have "put their back out" — they have not.
- They believe they have "slipped a disc" — they have not.
- They believe that, henceforth, life activities are going to be curtailed — they are not.

Let us examine each of these common misconceptions about back problems and, if possible, get rid of them.

Misconception One: The spine is a fragile thing.
The spine is not, despite its appearance, a precarious piling of various-sized vertebrae, one upon another, the whole sinuous contraption somehow held in an unstable vertical position by a complex of muscles and sinews.

It is widely believed that humankind's elevation from quadruped to biped is an aberration of nature that has left us with a weak link in our physiology — namely, the spine — thus disregarding the fact that many animals suffer back problems.

In fact, the spine is astonishingly durable and incredibly resilient under impact. Thousands of accident reports document victims' backs being subjected to enormous stresses without sustaining permanent injury.

If you think the spine is a fragile thing, watch a professional wrestling match on television. Beyond the fact that it is show-business rather than sport and that most of the pain is simulated, you cannot but be astonished when you see a 250-pound man fly through the air and crash to the canvas on his back without injury. Yes, the floor is padded, and, yes, it has been made resilient; nonetheless, the impact is enormous. Even more astonishing: these men do this kind of thing three or four times a week!

Let us labor the point:

You may have attended a rodeo and watched the broncho-busting or steer-wrestling. If you have, you have seen some of the most violent, teeth-jarring, spine-wrenching abuse it is possible to inflict on the human body. And yet, after being thrown or having subdued a steer two to three times their weight, these skinny, unprepossessing men get up, dust themselves off and get ready for the next encounter.

And if that doesn't convince you that a healthy spine is anything but fragile, watch professional football and note, even up in the stands, the popping of the leather!

Misconception Two: You can "put your back out."
Understand this clearly: the sudden onset of back pain you have endured did not result from your "putting your

back out." The spine doesn't, in anything short of a cataclysmic disaster, "go out."

The assumption many make when they endure a sharp pain in the back is that they have done something to cause one or more of the vertebrae to be forced out of line and that this is an extremely dangerous, even life-threatening occurrence. If this is your concern, set your mind at ease: the possibility of such a thing happening is remote in the extreme.

The simple fact is that, except in the most extraordinary circumstances, backs don't "go out." This misconception commonly worries first-time visitors to a chiropractor's office or others when they bend over first thing in the morning and hear a loud pop from the neck or back. Often, when the spine is manipulated by a chiropractor, you will hear a cracking sound. But, as any responsible practitioner will tell you, the sound has nothing to do with vertebrae slipping in or out of alignment; it results when a joint is suddenly forced slightly apart. A momentary vacuum is produced, the lubricating substance at the joint is vaporized, and the result is an audible pop.

To remind yourself of how insignificant the sound is, think back to when you were a child and used to amuse yourself and your friends by pulling on your fingers and popping your knuckles. Same thing with your back, and no more dangerous. The point is: you didn't "put your finger out" any more than you have "put your back out" when you hear similar sounds from that area.

It must be stated that people actually do break their backs. The term is a frightening one and usually creates the image of a fatal injury or permanent paralysis. The fact is, oddly enough, that a fracture of one of the vertebrae — if it does not damage the spinal cord — may produce nothing more than minor discomfort. If, however, you have hurt your back in a bad fall, don't dismiss it simply because you have full mobility in your legs and toes. Talk to your doctor. X-rays will reveal whether there is damage or not.

The pain you are feeling is not in your spine but in the muscles, ligaments and tendons that surround it and activate it. It is true that the vertebrae are subject to certain malformations as you age, and that these can sometimes be a source of pain. It is also true, as we shall see, that the discs in your spine can sustain injury and cause pain, but don't add to your problems by imagining that your pain is the result of some terrible misalignment of the vertebrae, that you have "put your back out" and that you are in serious jeopardy.

You haven't and you aren't.

Misconception Three: You have "slipped a disc."

Between most of the vertebrae are tough, resilient pads called discs. They serve two functions: they act as shock-absorbers and as joints of a sort, giving your spine flexibility. Each of these discs is securely encapsulated between two vertebrae and is exceedingly tough — so tough that, under compression, a healthy disc is stronger even than the bone of the vertebrae.

Discs have two components: a flexible outer layer called the *anulus fibrosis* and an inner substance called the *nucleus pulposis*, a gelatinous fluid, mostly water. Discs — like the rest of our body — are subject to wear and tear as we age. They dehydrate, lose some thickness and resiliency and can weaken, even rupture, and this can put pressure on nerves leading from the spinal column to various parts of the body. This slow deterioration does not, however, commonly lead to sudden back trauma but rather to a continuous low-grade discomfort ranging from numbness and tingling to chronic pain — the familiar "nagging backache."

The discs in the low back are, however, susceptible to injury, especially as the result of twisting motions (especially repeated twisting motions), usually when lifting, and can bulge or even rupture if seriously abused. And if the protrusion resulting from the rupture presses on a nerve, severe pain can result. Of all the aches to which the back is subject, a damaged disc can be among the most agonizing. Disc troubles lead to surgery more often than any other group of back problems.

But be assured: the chances of a ruptured disc happening to you are slight. It occurs in only 0.1 to 0.5 percent of men — most commonly men in their early thirties, seldom happening to men past fifty and even less frequently to women. If you had ruptured a disc you would have known immediately that something had gone wrong in your back. There is usually (but not necessarily immediately) intense pain, a numbness or weakness in one or both legs, and other, often dramatic symptoms.

If that is not your condition, don't brood about it.

Misconception Four: From this time forward, your activities are going to be seriously curtailed.
If what you are suffering is a typical acute back attack, it is likely — despite the intensity of the pain — that you will make a swift recovery, be back on your feet within days and be your old self within a few weeks. That's what happens 90 percent of the time. And having recovered, there is no reason why you should not be able to resume your normal participation in a full range of activities, from work, to active sports, to having sex.

There is a factor that could hinder your recovery and turn your episode of back trouble into a lifelong problem. That factor is *you.*

Having offered reassurances that you have not "put your back out" or "slipped a disc" or permanently injured yourself or condemned yourself to a curtailed lifestyle, let us impress upon you that the greatest threat to your recovery is your reaction to your problem.

An episode of back trauma, either neglected or magnified out of proportion, can lead to a life of chronic back pain and to attacks much more serious than the one you are enduring.

You will get over this current attack if you act sensibly, but your full and permanent recovery is up to you. So have a stern little talk with yourself in which you remind yourself of three things:

- Your doctor's reassurance that your back problem is not the result of a physical abnormality or serious injury or disease is not a subterfuge to postpone giving you the bad news, but is a fact.
- The pain you are enduring will be short-lived. It will pass and you will, *sooner than you think at the moment*, be back to normal.
- Your most urgent task is to banish your unreasonable fears, ease your tension and commit yourself to a program of rehabilitation that will make unlikely a repetition of this bout with pain.

The failure to do this can lead to a condition known as chronic back pain. It is by no means common but neither is it rare, and such is the number of backaches in the general population that even a small percentage comprises a large number.

Chronic back pain appears to be a residual illness. Its victims originally suffered an attack of acute back pain but did not, as is normal, recover from it within a period of a few weeks or months. Instead, the pain hangs on and becomes the dominant reality in the individual's life.

In fact, there is no clearly isolatable reason for the pain other than the pain itself. The patient is not simply malingering, nor is the pain imaginary; it is real and varies in intensity. Nor will it do simply to dismiss the pain as psychological, although there can be little doubt that it proceeds from the patient's psyche and not primarily from the site of the distress. The pain can sometimes be eased with medication but, more often than not, the drug becomes a part of the illness and intensifies the problem. The same is true when alcohol becomes the palliative.

All of which emphasizes the importance of keeping your back problem in perspective. It has come, it hurts and it is inconvenient, but in all probability it will go. And life will be normal again.

If you find yourself increasingly brooding about your injury and discouraged, bestir yourself. Occupy your mind elsewhere — with books or television or friends or work. Make notes about challenges at work or in your family life, or things to be done when you are up and about again. Keep a daily log in which you note what you do that day. Record the relative easing of the pain, the progress you are making in your exercises, the amount of time spent out of bed.

After a few days, go back and review your notes; you will be bound to recognize the improvement.

5

Getting Comfortable in Bed

LET'S BEGIN THINKING ABOUT YOUR RECOVERY and about how soon you can get out of bed.

Following an attack of severe back pain, getting back on your feet is no simple matter of saying, "Guess I'll get up now." In fact, after you have essayed a few vain attempts, you may be more likely to say, "Maybe I'll wait a day or two."

There are no inflexible rules about how long your stay in bed should be. It depends in large part on how seriously you have injured your back, the kind of shape you are in and the type of individual you are. If, however, you have been in bed for a period of a month or more with little significant improvement, it is unlikely that bed rest is going to improve your condition. Consult with your doctor.

If this is your first attack, presumably you have already checked with your doctor. If you are an old hand, however, the symptoms will be familiar and you will know by the character and the location of your pain whether or not this is a more serious attack than usual.

DON'T BE A LAYABOUT

Presuming that there is nothing organically wrong with your back, realize from the beginning that lying in bed any longer than necessary is bad for you. The longer you stay in bed the longer it will take to recover fully when you get back on your feet.

There is a rough rule of thumb: *each day spent in inactivity will require four to six days to return unused muscles to their previous tone.* Therefore, don't let fear or irresolution or moderate pain confine you to bed any longer than necessary.

So, after the first two or three days (or longer; it's a judgment-call only you can make), you must begin to weigh the amount of discomfort in your back against the deterioration of muscle-tone in the rest of your body.

Bear in mind, of course, that any injured muscle should be rested, occasionally immobilized, until the inflammation and the swelling have diminished. That is why an individual with a badly sprained ankle is put on crutches and why a broken bone is put in a cast. The body's natural healing processes must be given the opportunity to work, and a premature attempt to return to normal activity can prove worse than becoming a layabout.

THE BENEFITS OF BED REST

You will find it easy to understand why resting your injured back is essential if you consider the mechanics related to body posture. When you stand erect, your spine and the related muscles in the injured area take

100 percent of the strain. When you lie down, that figure immediately reduces to 25 percent.

Bed rest has a further advantage: the reduction of the load on the injured back muscles will help avoid a recurrence of the body's response to a muscle sprain in the back — namely, spasm in the surrounding muscles. If you are still subject to the occasional muscle spasm, staying put will help avoid or minimize it.

In most cases, you really don't need an expert to tell you when to get off your back and back on your feet; your body will inform you. Use this as a basis for your judgment:

• If getting up hurts but is bearable, get up.
• If getting up hurts a lot, stay put.

Don't, for any reason, aggravate the injury, but don't be unduly self-protective.

GETTING COMFORTABLE

Priority Number One is, of course, to get comfortable. And that can be a real problem.

You may normally relish extending your "sack time" on weekends and may believe at times that you can never get too much of it. But the body is not accustomed to life on the horizontal and it will soon become clear that prolonged bed rest can become too much of a good thing.

That is especially true when you are in bed after an acute attack because your affliction seriously restricts your movement.

Know before you begin trying to get comfortable that there is no "best position." The rule is: *assume any position that is less uncomfortable than the other positions*. Do not, however, make the mistake of limiting yourself to one position — even if that one is relatively pain-free and changing to others might produce pain. To lie immobilized for extended periods will produce stiffness and soreness in muscles other than the affected ones, and that is the path to increasing discomfort. As we will see later, you should be exercising all your muscles except those in your back.

Lying on your back

The two positions most likely to produce some easing of your pain are:

1. on your back with a pillow under your knees and
2. on your side in the so-called fetal position.

Most of the time, the most comfortable position is on the back with a firm pillow under the knees. Some prefer two or even three pillows — experimenting will tell you what is best for you. The purpose of the pillow is twofold: to stretch the lower-back muscles and to keep you from arching your back.

By placing a pillow under the knees you achieve a modified "pelvic tilt" — a flattening of the arch of the lower back and a forward tilt of the pelvic region.

This posture is beneficial because the muscles in the area of an injury tend to contract in order to immobilize the injured muscles. It is a form of damage-control by your autonomic nervous system, a reflex action, the purpose of which is to protect the injured muscles from further injury. Gently stretching your lower-back muscles helps keep them from constricting, possibly going into spasm.

There is no fixed rule about the placement of the pillow(s) or about its bulk. Some prefer a support no more bulky than a rolled-up bath towel. Experiment. You may, for instance, find it better to position the pillow beneath your thighs, just above the knees. Settle for what works.

Supporting your head

It is important that the pillow under your head not be bulky. Use one that supports your head in a position that more or less duplicates the normal relationship of your head to your neck and shoulders when standing. A too-thick pillow under your head may intensify the pain in your back and add to it a pain in the neck.

Incidentally, the pillow you use under your head while lying on your side should be thicker than the one you use when lying on your back. The objective in both positions is to keep your head and neck aligned with your back in the same general relationship they are in when you are standing.

Though you may normally sleep on a foam-rubber pillow, you might be well advised to switch to the conventional feather-filled variety during your recuperation. A foam pillow gives pliant support but it tends to be "active," rolling your head rather than letting it settle in. Again, do what works for you. You may even wish to try lying with no pillow at all, or with only a rolled bath-towel under your neck.

This is hardly the moment to go shopping, but a variety of contoured "orthopedic" pillows have come onto the market, and some find them helpful. They come in different shapes and sizes and are designed to reverse what commonly happens when you use a conventional pillow.

When lying on a conventional pillow that is too bulky or too unresilient, the head is tilted forward and the neck is left unsupported. This position can quickly induce pain in the back of the neck and shoulders. Lying on your side, there will often be an unsupported gap between your head and shoulder, which can put a strain on the cervical muscles on one side of the neck.

So-called orthopedic pillows have been developed to counter these problems. They are made of foam rubber — firmer than most foam-rubber pillows — and have a raised, rounded configuration on the lower edge to support the neck as well as the head. Different types are made for sleeping on the side and on the back. Some find them uncomfortable. Others — especially those subject to neck pain — recommend them highly. Before you commit yourself, try one overnight, leaving the protective plastic cover on so that you may return it if you are not satisfied. They are not expensive.

Lying on your side

Another way to make yourself relatively comfortable is to turn onto your side. The actions required to do this may briefly increase your pain but will do you no harm.

Incidentally, one of the fundamental benefits of bed rest is the reassuring knowledge that, while you may endure sustained discomfort and the occasional sharp pain, you are in no danger of doing yourself further injury. Your bed is a safe haven. You are not yet out of the woods but you are on the path that will get you there. Let this knowledge help you to relax.

To move onto your side (presuming that you are on your back), half draw up your knees, one at a time. Place your right hand on your chest (to get it out of the way) and extend your left arm so that you may start your upper body moving to the right by pushing down on the bed. Now, in one unhurried, coordinated motion, simply roll onto your side.

It is important to keep your legs and torso aligned as the turn is made. Do not twist.

If your bed is soft and you are in a kind of hollow, you may find it difficult to roll over. You can solve this problem by turning slightly to the right and extending your left arm vertically. Then, maintaining that position, bring your arm and your knees over as you roll onto your right side. The weight of your arm as it descends will help bring your shoulders over.

Again, *do not twist*. Maintain your body as a unit.

To return to lying on your back, resume the fetal position and stretch out your right arm. Now, in a single, coordinated move, keeping your knees together, press on the bed with your arm and roll slowly to the left. Once again, maintain your torso and bent legs as a unit.

The fetal position

Having made the move to lie on your side, you are now in what is commonly called the fetal position — your back gently curved, your knees bent, your arms crooked loosely in front of your chest. Next to lying on your back, a pillow under your knees, this is undoubtedly the most relaxing position available to you.

Do not strain unduly to draw your knees high. Adjust them, one at a time, to where you feel most at ease.

You will find it advantageous to place a pillow between your knees. It will keep the pelvis aligned. You may discover, however, that while the usual bed pillow is comfortable, it is too resilient and too insulating. Almost certainly, it will make the insides of your thighs perspire. If it does, substitute a less-bulky cushion.

Remember that "a change is as good as a rest," and if, after a while, you become stiff or generally uncomfortable in the fetal position, you can vary it by straightening one or the other leg, forming a kind of figure-four with your legs. Do it slowly the first time. You will then have the feel of it.

Lying on your stomach

The one position you should be careful about is lying on your stomach. It may normally be your favorite position for sleep but, in the circumstances, it could prove painful. The normal sag in the bed at mid-point will increase the curvature of your spine and produce a sway-back.

And, depending on the nature of your injury, that could sharply increase your pain.

Lying on the stomach also has the disadvantage of requiring you to turn your neck to one side.

If this is your first back attack and you don't yet know the cause, avoid lying on your stomach until your doctor has made a diagnosis. If you insist on trying it, take it slowly. You may find it very relaxing. First, however, remove the pillow from beneath your head and place a thin pillow or a cushion beneath your midriff.

It should be obvious that none of the moves we have been describing can be accomplished unless the blankets are first pushed out of the way or loosely tented about your body. If they aren't, you may conclude the move and find yourself entangled in the bedclothes.

IT'S EITHER TOO HOT OR TOO COLD

If you find yourself alternating between being too warm and too cold (not unlikely because you will be taking medication and, as well, your emotions will be switching between apprehension and relief), don't simply push the blankets down. Have your spouse or a friend free the bottom of the blankets, leaving only the sheet tucked in. You can then flip individual blankets aside when you get too warm and flip them back into position without calling for assistance.

This is important because, if, seeking to cool off, you push the covers down, you may be unable to reach them when you need to. Bending forward to retrieve them could cause severe pain. If there is no one available to help and you find yourself too warm, flip the upper portion of the blankets aside as best you can, but leave them within reach.

EATING IN BED

If your back is very painful, eating in bed may be difficult for the first day or two, and no simple thing after that.

If sitting up to eat is too risky, stay with liquids, drinking them from the spout of a small teapot or, if you happen to have one, an old-fashioned mustache-cup. There are many kinds of nutritious soups available and a great variety of juices. With sandwiches or cold cuts — or other foods that won't drip and mess the bed — you can easily satisfy your hunger.

And remember the old saying: "Fingers were made before forks."

There is an alternative to sitting up to eat: try lying on your side. The tray can be placed on the bed within easy reach, and you can see how you make out one-handed. A word of caution: take care not to prop yourself up too high or to stay there too long; a lateral strain on the spine could be painful.

You should not delay any longer than necessary moving into a sitting position to eat. Once you have passed the time when such a move is filled with jeopardy, try to accomplish it. You are the best judge of when you can manage it. Go to neither extreme: don't lie transfixed by fear but, conversely, don't do the macho bit to demonstrate your stoic qualities.

When you are ready, have the person who prepares your food arrange two or three pillows more or less diagonally against the head of the bed. Bring your knees up and, easing your body weight with your feet and arms, work your upper back and shoulders onto the pillows. Make certain, when you are finally in position, that there is support for the small of your back.

Once settled in, put a pillow under your knees — ideally a firm and bulky one. It will keep you from sliding down. More important, it will tilt your pelvis forward and thus flatten the arch of your back.

Balance the tray on a pillow. Keep the first session brief and, when you return to lying flat, you will feel good about yourself. Your appetite will have been satisfied and you will have taken an important step toward returning to the world of the vertical.

6

Organizing the Sickroom

INASMUCH AS YOU ARE GOING TO SPEND A CONSID-
erable amount of time in bed for the next few days,
organize your world.

It is a very circumscribed world, and there you are, at
the center of it, virtually immobilized. You can't be forever calling out to others for one thing or another, so get
organized.

If you don't, you will soon get on everybody's nerves.

There will be many things you can't do for yourself and
you will have no option *but* to seek help. However, with a
little planning, you can greatly reduce your demands on
others.

THE BED ITSELF
You are going to spend the next few days in your bed:
sleep in it, sit in it, eat in it, read in it, entertain in it,
watch television in it, exercise in it and even take care of
your bodily functions while in it — so you should adapt it
to your needs as much as possible, as soon as possible.

As for the bed itself: it is unlikely that your sick-bed will be other than the one you and your spouse normally sleep in; in which case you will have to make do as best you can. If, however, it is a poor, spavined thing, sagging in the middle, and enough in itself to give you a bad back, some action may have to be taken. Not to do so could greatly increase your discomfort and delay your recovery.

Optimum sack time

When you realize that you spend one-third of your life in bed (eight of each twenty-four hours — *twenty-five years* if you live to age seventy-five!), it is astonishing that so many people give so little thought to the bed they sleep in.

But, if you are subject to frequent or chronic back pain, it is imperative that you give the matter serious consideration and, if it seems necessary, make an investment in your rest.

Begin by realizing that there is no one "best" mattress. There are, however, good and bad mattresses in varying degrees, and some serious shortcomings in some.

The most important consideration is this: *don't sleep on a mattress that sags.*

All but the cheapest contemporary mattresses are built with coiled springs designed to conform to the contours of your body. They rest on a "boxspring" and are unlike the old-fashioned mattress, which turned into a kind of metal hammock when you lay on it. Nonetheless, despite all the modern improvements, inexpensive mattresses (or mattresses that have been used over a period of years) tend to develop hollows or permanent indentations that are anything but supportive of injured back muscles. One of their worst features is that they make it difficult to change position, and inasmuch as it is desirable to do this often, this drawback can lead to pain in the back or joints come morning.

The problem may be considerably worsened if your bed partner weighs much more than you do.

Your back is not a fragile thing, but hours of distorted "posture" night after night can strain your neck and back and cause you to begin your day with stiff or sore muscles, which by virtue of this stiffness, may be more subject to injury.

Sleeping in a sling

It is widely believed that a hammock is the ideal place in which to relax. And it is true that, for an hour or two on a lazy day, the motion can induce a soporific state. However, it is anything but the ideal repository for an ailing back and illustrates perfectly why a sagging mattress can be hazardous to your health.

The navies of the world once slept their men in hammocks, but the armed services have never been noted for their concern about making life easy for enlistees (note that the captain slept in a bunk). The hammock's usefulness afloat derived mostly from the fact that it dampened the transfer of the motion of the ship and thus countered seasickness. Even more important, in the confined space aboard a ship, it could quickly be unslung and stored.

Despite its appeal, a hammock may be one of the worst places in the world to rest an ailing back. And a mattress that sags is nearly as bad.

Bed and board

If your mattress is suspect but you can't afford a new one, at least improve the one you are sleeping on by placing a board beneath it.

You can buy a sheet of $3/4''$ plywood at any lumberyard. Have it cut to size, and place it between the mattress and the boxspring. This simple change can do much to minimize the "morning backache" you may have been enduring.

If your spouse is adamantly opposed to "sleeping on a board," position the plywood only on your side. Unfortunately, if the bed sags significantly, you may find your side tilted toward the center and be forced to combat the tendency to roll to the middle of the bed. In such circumstances, a blanket folded lengthwise or a strategically positioned pillow or two may be your only recourse. Place the blanket or pillow beneath the edge of the board toward the center of the bed. It will at least minimize the tilt. (Incidentally, if your spouse is that indifferent to your discomfort, you may have chanced upon the psychological reason for your back trouble.)

There is no perfect bed, but some beds are better than others. The only fundamental requirement is that the mattress provide support through the length of your body. A rule of thumb might be: better too firm than too soft. However, if the insertion of a plywood sheet gives you the feeling of sleeping on the board itself, you may wish to add a foam-rubber or down- filled underpad. An Australian "Wool-rest" mattress cover is expensive but worth the investment.

The waterbed
There are many who favor a waterbed. There can be no doubt that the waterbed does conform better to the body and therefore better distributes the support. It offers a further advantage: the water in the mattress can be heated, and this can contribute to relaxation.

Early waterbeds were little more than flat containers of water, and the slightest movement of a bedmate could set up swells and wavelets that could almost produce *mal de mer*. The contemporary waterbed uses baffles to minimize this transferred motion and also offers better distributed support.

In the final analysis, the choice of a waterbed over a well-constructed conventional mattress becomes a matter of personal preference. Arguments can be made for the superiority of one over the other. Neither is demonstrably superior to the other for a given individual.

Before you buy, test. There are waterbed stores that offer a money-back guarantee, but installing and removing a waterbed is no simple matter. Water is non-condensable and is therefore heavy. The mattress takes time to fill and even more time to come to room temperature. The mattress itself requires a special base, so give it careful thought before you commit.

If you are intent on a "trial-run," many metropolitan hotels (and not a few tourist cabins) have rooms with waterbeds, and some will rent you a room for a few hours at a "day rate," permitting you to try the mattress out. Don't be surprised, however, if the desk clerk seems slightly skeptical about your reasons for wanting such a brief occupancy. He's heard such explanations before.

The futon bed

The Japanese system for sleeping is growing in popularity, and you may wish to investigate it. It was introduced in the West some years ago in the form of the futon bed — essentially, a mattress to be placed on the floor — and has had a considerable vogue, especially among health addicts and the young. There are now elaborate and expensive versions of the beds, some incorporating a variety of exotic features such as dozens of small magnets in the bedcover (it is argued that they are health-inducing), duvets, variations in mattress texture and special molded pillows of the kind commonly sold in stores specializing in serving people with back problems.

The futon has much to commend it, and you may wish to investigate the possibilities.

What to wear in bed

Early on during your enforced bed rest, give thought to what you will wear — and we are here discussing comfort and convenience rather than style.

The usual pajamas or nightgown are impractical. As you change position in bed — and you will be doing a lot of this — they become twisted, bunched and binding. And because such bed attire can be awkward, even painful to adjust when you can't easily arch or twist your body, it can become the source of considerable discomfort.

The best solution is to wear nothing. If you are not disposed to lie naked between the sheets, wear your underwear. If you prefer to keep your torso covered — for reasons of modesty or because the room is cold — a T-shirt or a shortie-nightgown will serve admirably. Particularly useful is a T-shirt with the lower part cut away 8 to 10 inches below the sleeve insert. It keeps the shoulders covered but doesn't get twisted when you turn.

THE TELEPHONE: YOUR OUTER-WORLD CONNECTION

If there is no telephone in your bedroom, rig an extension cord from the phone jack in a nearby room. If necessary, get two cords and string them down the stairs or along the hallway. Extension cords are inexpensive and, in the circumstances, well worth the few dollars of outlay. They are available in any hardware store. A cellular phone is, of course, the ideal solution.

Inasmuch as you are going to be bedridden for the next few days, the telephone is indispensable. It will enable you to:

- consult with your doctor,
- communicate with friends,

- order from stores that deliver,
- keep in touch with the office,
- do business with clients, and
- accomplish any number of tasks.

First thing in the morning, have the telephone placed within reach on the night table or on the bed. It is your connection to the outside world and it will prove invaluable if your confinement drags on.

Friends will be calling to ask how you are, and it will lessen the demands on your spouse if you take the calls. (With a bedridden patient in the house, your spouse will have more than enough to do.) Any time you don't feel up to a telephone conversation, you can easily transfer the responsibility, or pull the plug.

Telephone calls — coming in or going out at your option — will help pass the long, inactive days and get your mind off yourself — *no small thing!*

Beyond that, because your emotional reactions may be slightly abnormal, the telephone will give you a sense of security when members of the family are away from the house and you are alone. It is astonishing how easily a victim of a back attack can work up a considerable panic, imagining a seizure while in the bathroom or elsewhere with no one available to help.

THE BOX AND THE BOOK

When you are confined to bed for even a brief period, time moves on leaden feet. The days, and sometimes the nights, are long, and boredom becomes a burden. There are any number of things you can do to move the time along.

If there isn't a television set in the bedroom — and these days that's almost an exception to the rule — have the set brought in from the living room — unless, of course, it's a billboard-size monster. If that isn't feasible, portable television sets can be rented locally by the day or week. Check your yellow pages.

Daytime television is largely a wasteland but it is better than staring at the ceiling or lying there contemplating your misery.

So have the TV set up in the bedroom, if possible, placed higher than you would normally so that you don't have to bend your neck or prop yourself up to view the screen. This position could aggravate your back muscles. It may also produce stiffness in the neck and a surprising amount of soreness in the eyeballs.

If you are a TV addict and want to watch the tube even while resting on your side, prop a hand-mirror against a pillow, so angled that the screen is visible. Often, the mirror on the inside of a closet door can be so angled that the television screen is reflected there. The print in the commercials will read backwards, but count this a bonus.

You can further speed the reluctant hours by reading.

Because you may be reading more than usual (including the daily newspapers — from the front page to the obituaries!), arrange an adequate light source. Tilt the shade on the night-table lamp or, better, rig a gooseneck or clamp-on light at the head of the bed. A good source of illumination will minimize eyestrain and keep you from twisting your body into uncomfortable positions, trying to get enough light onto the page.

You will soon discover that prolonged reading while lying down isn't pure pleasure. Because you are flat on your back, your arms will soon tire from the need to hold the printed material high. So will your neck.

Prop pillows beneath your elbows. Change the book from hand to hand. A simple elastic band will serve to keep the pages open while you are one-handing it. Try extending your arms vertically for a while or even lying on your side. Reading while more or less flat on your back can quickly tire you but, beyond the benefits reading yields, it is worth the effort if it does no more than get your mind off yourself and help pass the day.

Nobody promised you a rose garden.

If you are one of those commited types who want to improve each shining hour, you can catch up on your serious reading by getting in touch with your local bookstore. Most bookstores and many public libraries now have some of the classics and a selection of contemporary bestsellers available on audio-cassettes.

If you want to work, use a clipboard and a pencil — a pencil because, as you will learn, ballpoint and conventional pens run dry when held business-end upwards. If you don't have a clipboard, substitute two shirt cardboards, with a paperclip to bind them together and keep the notepaper in place. If you are lying flat, stand the clipboard upright on a pillow placed on your chest; it will help you avoid eye- and neck-strain.

VISITORS WELCOME

Encourage visitors. Not least, their presence will move the clock along and will help get your mind off your plight.

As well, a visitor will give you an audience to play to.

Back-pain sufferers are justly renowned for their willingness to talk about their affliction. You will have a particularly delightful time if your visitor has never had a back problem — there is so much suffering to describe, so much sympathy to be elicited and such a variety of problems to be detailed.

Your joy may be alloyed, however, if your guest is a back-pain veteran who can match you symptom for symptom and go on to overwhelm you with the variety of exotic treatments he or she has undertaken.

You will want to put a time limit on visitors. Inasmuch as they are likely to sit in one place, you will soon find yourself uncomfortable or suffering pain in the neck from continually looking in their direction. Moreover, what may be enjoyable for you can quickly become a burden to your spouse, who will be overworked as it is and may come to resent running snacks and refreshments back and forth from the kitchen.

7

Exercise without Movement

ONE OF THE PROBLEMS RELATED TO BEING IMMO-
bilized after an acute back attack is that the muscles of
the rest of your body begin a swift deterioration.

Consequently, it is fundamentally important that you
not remain in bed any longer than necessary and that
you do not permit your muscles to deteriorate from lack of
use. Muscular strength is increased through exercise;
unused muscles quickly lose tone and grow slack.

But, with the initial pain fresh in your memory and
with the overriding concern that you may bring on another back attack if you make an unwise move, the temptation will be strong to leave bad enough alone and to
postpone any avoidable movement that might create
problems.

It is important to overcome any undue apprehension in
this matter, not least because tension was probably a
major contributor to the original attack. Fretting about
the possibility of a recurrence can itself contribute to a
recurrence.

There are two immediate and equally important challenges before you then: to diminish your apprehension and to begin to work actively on your recovery.

Fortunately, there is a system of exercises that will maintain good muscle tone while requiring virtually no movement and thus little risk. It is called isometrics.

MUSCLE VERSUS MUSCLE

Isometrics (*iso* = same, *metric* = length) is a system of exercises that, rather than depend on strenuous activity, pits one muscle against another (or against an immovable object) in an intense but motionless pushing, pulling, pressing or flexing. To put it simply: isometrics is the tensing of a muscle against unyielding resistance. Many of the elaborate machines in today's muscle factories employ the principle. Most of the serious body-builders use it to shape their physiques. It is not the ideal system if your goal is to become limber and flexible, but it is unexcelled for building strength and increasing muscle tone.

When you are bedridden and must remain reasonably quiescent, isometrics has the virtue of maintaining muscle tone and strength while requiring no movement. You can do it while flat on your back simply by opposing your muscles with your muscles.

To understand the essential principle, hold your arms across your chest, clasp your hands and pull equally with both arms. There is no movement involved, but you will feel the muscles of your shoulders and upper arms contract and grow rigid.

Now, reverse the process. Place the palms of your hands flat against each other and push. You'll feel the result in your upper arms and chest.

Now that the principle is clear (you oppose one muscle with another, moving neither), let us proceed through a series of simple exercises designed to maintain a degree of muscular fitness without having to move your body and thus produce pain in your back.

At the end of each exercise, relax briefly before going on to the next. During this first session you may wish to do each exercise only once. When you feel ready, repeat each one three times before moving to the next.

Upper-body exercise without movement

1. *Repeat the exercises described above*, using as much force as seems wise. Hold for a slow count of five (one thousand, two thousand, three thousand, etc.) and then release.
2. *Extend your arms straight out from your chest* (vertically, inasmuch as you are lying on your back). Place your palms together and exert pressure. You will feel this in your chest and shoulders, but also in the muscles of your upper back. Your arms in the same position, lock your hands and, this time, pull outward for the usual count of five, then release.
3. *Raise your outstretched arms above your head.* Place the palms of your hands against each other and push. Now, lock your fingers and pull. Hold each for a count of five, then release.
4. *Stetch your arms sideways so that your body forms a cross.* Now, using the bed as resistance, press down. Hold for a count of five, then release.
5. *Place your arms alongside the body* and press with both hands simultaneously against the sides of the thighs. Now, arms in the same position, press down against the bed. Hold and release.
6. *Place your right upper arm on the bed alongside your chest, with the forearm bent vertical.* Reach across with the left hand and clasp your hands. Now do a curl with the bent arm while resisting with the other. Use some caution; you could feel it in your low

back, but don't be too easily deterred. Hold for five, then change arms and repeat.

7. *To strengthen the neck muscles*, place the palm of your right hand against the side of your head and push. Resist the pressure with your neck muscles so that no movement takes place. Repeat with the left hand. Place a hand against your brow and resist as you try to lift your head. Finish by pressing your head back into the pillow. Doing this, keep your chin tucked in. (Take care to use only moderate pressure in all of these neck exercises; your neck muscles may not be fit and you could strain rather than strengthen them.)

Lower-body exercise

None of the upper-body exercises described above should produce any pain of consequence. There may be some, but it will be minimal, so persevere. Working on the lower body adds a degree of jeopardy, but even if you feel a twinge or two, don't give up; simply ease off for a day or two. In the highly unlikely event that the pain is severe, stop immediately.

1. *Begin to work on your lower body by learning the pelvic tilt.* The pelvic tilt is not an isometric exercise but is *the basic exercise for people with trouble-prone backs*. If you have never learned to do it, turn to page 181.

   Its primary purpose is to strengthen the muscles of the stomach. This is important because abused and unused muscles tend to diminish in resiliency and thus become more subject to injury.

   It relieves pressure on the facet joints; this is important because they are the stabilizing "hinges" of the back and crucial when you bend over or straighten up.

It strengthens the abdominal muscles. This is important because strong stomach muscles are essential in maintaining the back at vertical and as supplementary power in bending, lifting, etc. Strive to make the pelvic tilt as normal as breathing. Not only will it improve your posture, it will protect you from many an episode of back pain.

2. *To strengthen the inside of the thighs*, put your feet together and press them against each other. Hold for a count of five and release.

3. *To strengthen the outsides of the thigh muscles*, cross your legs at the ankles, hook your feet on each other and push your legs outward. Do not bend the knees.

There are are many other appropriate isometric exercises. Do some experimenting. One word of caution: begin each exercise guardedly. Be neither reckless nor timid. If a specific exercise produces a jab of pain in your back, ease off for a day or two.

One of the attendant benefits of isometric exercises during the early stages of recovery is the fact that, when you are back on your feet, you will find that you are making more than the usual demands on your arms and shoulders. The exercises described above will prepare you to handle them. Even more important, they will help hasten your return to normal.

LEARNING TO RELAX

Your doctor may prescribe an analgesic or a tranquilizer. The first is for the affected muscles; the second is for your state of mind. Well and good, but there is much you can do yourself to diminish such tension as you may feel.

Fix this firmly in your consciousness: *tension is the enemy*. Unless you learn to handle it, you are almost certainly going to be bedeviled by recurrent bouts of back pain. Handling tension is discussed in detail in Chapter 18. You may wish to turn to it now.

8

Back on Your Feet

YOU HAVE BEEN BEDRIDDEN FOR A FEW DAYS, possibly a few weeks. It is now time to rejoin the world of the vertical.

You may have already postponed getting up longer than you should have or, conversely, may be so itchy to get back on your feet that you are pushing things. It is impossible to offer blind counsel on the timing; no one can know the answer but you. It can be said, however, that if you have been sitting up in bed and making the various moves needed to turn over, eat, read or watch television without muscle spasm or strong pain, you are ready to give it a try.

Before you begin, expect some discomfort, perhaps a twinge or two of pain and some weakness in your muscles. This is to be expected, so don't let it deter you.

If, however, the movement required to get up causes sharp pain, stay where you are for a day or two and then try again.

NO BIG DEAL

Three moves are used in getting out of bed. Described in detail, they sound complicated. In the doing, they combine into one smooth sequence of actions, as simple as those required to rise from a chair. We will detail them here because any major body movement shortly after a back attack is fraught with tension and touched with fear, and you will want all the information and reassurance you can get.

There is nothing to worry about. If you aren't ready to get up, you will quickly know it. If you are, you will find the requisite moves easier than you anticipate.

Before you begin, throw the sheets clear. Otherwise you may get tangled in them, hindering your movement and unnecessarily complicating the task.

STEP BY STEP

Prepare to get up by lying on your back. The first objective is to get your body turned diagonally toward the edge of the bed. We assume, in this description, that you are getting up on the left side of the bed. Bend your knees and put your hands beside the pelvic area. Elevate your buttocks slightly and angle them toward the edge of the mattress. Finish by hanging the lower half of your left leg over the edge. In making the move, you may find it helpful to elevate your hips with your hands.

Now, place both hands on the bed at waist height, elbows angled out from your body. Transferring most of your weight onto your left elbow and pushing with your right arm, raise your torso partially upright. As you come up, straighten your left arm, bringing your torso upright and simultaneously lowering your right leg over the edge of the bed as the turn is completed.

You are now seated on the side of the bed, both feet on the floor, much of your upper-body weight supported by your arms.

Do not remain there; the edge of the mattress can be an unstable seat. Bring your feet close to the bed, slide your buttocks to the edge of the mattress and, leaning forward slightly, stand up. On your feet, straighten up slowly.

Describing each move makes it sound complicated, but it's not. *It is actually a single, coordinated movement.*

Two helpful hints:

1. Form your hands into fists before you begin. This lengthens your arms and makes the lifting easier.
2. Don't twist your torso. Keep it in line with your hips, maintaining your upper body as a unit.

The lift into the sitting position takes effort, of course, because your arm muscles may have weakened during your time in bed. But don't concern yourself about it; it is well within your ability.

Don't stay on your feet too long the first time up. And before you move away from the bed, use the first thirty seconds to massage your lower back. The muscles will be stiff and weaker than normal. A firm but gentle massage will relax them.

Take a leisurely stroll about the house but don't overdo it. And don't try the stairs unless there's a handrail and you have no doubt that you can negotiate them, up *and* down.

GETTING BACK INTO BED

When you begin to tire, get back in bed. Doing so is almost a reversal of the process of getting out — only simpler.

Stand with your back to the bed, about mid-way, turned diagonally, so that the back of your right leg is touching the mattress and so positioned that when you lie down your head will end up on the pillow.

Now, sit down, *taking most of the weight on your arms, the hands formed into fists.* Then, simply continuing the motion without a break, let your body roll back until you are lying on the bed with your head on the pillow. Do it without tension and without twisting, completely relaxed. The best description of the movement is that it is a *controlled, slow-motion fall.*

Once you're down, make yourself comfortable.

You will undoubtedly feel some fatigue after your initial out-of-bed foray and the bed will be a welcome place. But, more important, your spirit will be buoyed up by the achievement and the realization that you have taken a significant stride toward recovery.

9

Tub or Shower?

THE ACUTE PHASE OF YOUR BACK ATTACK HAS eased. Now comes the recovery period, and its early days can be filled with challenges.

Confined to your bed, you have been largely dependent on others. Back on your feet, you must regain your independence and deal with such mundane tasks as bathing, getting dressed, meeting your minimal daily obligations and taking care of your body's needs.

You discover that familiar rituals have suddenly become worrisome problems. You find yourself debating such things as:

- whether your back is up to the leaning over required to shampoo your hair and do your makeup,
- whether, rather than shave, you should use this opportunity to grow a beard,
- whether, rather than tub or shower, you can make do with a sponge-bath,

- whether you should face the problems of getting dressed or just lounge about in a bathrobe or housecoat.

Even such mundane matters as the condition of your bowels and whether or not to take a laxative can become matters of concern.

For these reasons and others, it is important as well as beneficial to bathe as soon as is reasonably possible. After days and nights in the sometimes sweaty, twisted sheets, one's outlook can bottom out. Nothing can raise the spirits more and kindle optimism better than a hot bath or shower.

TO BATHE OR TO SHOWER?

In the tentative first days out of bed it is astonishing how intimidating the prospect of, say, taking a bath can be. You can become so hypersensitive to the slightest twinge of pain, so apprehensive about having a spasm while getting into or out of the tub, so concerned about being unable to straighten up after bending over the bathroom sink, that your daily cleanliness routines can be transformed from a time of refreshment into an ordeal.

It need not be so.

There are ways to go about these essentially simple tasks that can remove the risk and transform them into the high point of your day.

Taking a shower

In the days immediately following an acute attack, a shower is much preferable to a bath. This is so because the shower can be undertaken with less effort and less risk and because it offers supplementary benefits. In addition to cleansing your body, you can shampoo your hair and, while you are at it, administer a massage to the affected muscles of your back.

Despite all these advantages, the shower has its hazards, and they must be borne in mind.

If there is not a skid-proof mat on the bottom of the tub, forgo it. Your sense of balance may be impaired by your concern about the vulnerability of your back, and your ability to concentrate on what you are about may be less than usual. One slip and you could go down. And because it has no soft surfaces, the bathroom is a dangerous place in which to take a fall.

Refreshment in the shower

A shower stall is the ideal place in which to bathe and in which to relax your sore muscles.

You can go into it without risk. Its four walls are at hand for support. The floor tiles are usually nonskid and are being flushed free of soap by the flow from the shower head. The soap-holder is within easy reach; there is no need to stress your back by bending over.

There are, nonetheless, certain preparations to be made before you begin. Check that there is soap in the holder, and no more than one bar. If there is none, you will have to go dripping from the shower to fetch some. If there are two bars, you are liable, occupied with washing, to return the one you are using to the holder and have both fall to the floor.

It is not uncommon to drop the soap while showering, especially when the bar has become reduced in size from use. Bending over to retrieve it — especially if your eyes are closed against the suds — can lead to blind gropings while crouched low on the floor, and that can be extremely risky.

An ideal solution is the so-called soap-on-a-rope. When using it, take the precaution of giving the rope a turn about your wrist to ensure that it won't slip off. When not in use, it can be hung from your neck within easy reach. If you wish merely to have it handy, hang it on the pipe leading to the shower head.

In many stall-showers, the device that reroutes the water from the spigot to the shower head is close to the floor. Bending down to activate it is unnecessary. Fashion a simple tool by flattening a common wire coat hanger so that the hook is at one end. The hook can then be used to pull the lever that routes the flow to the shower head. Between showers, hang it from one of the faucet heads.

Take the opportunity while in the shower to shampoo your hair. It is much more convenient and considerably safer than doing it at the sink. The lathering is easier and the rinsing more thorough. All important: you don't have to bend over while doing it.

If you find it stressful to lean over the sink to shave, try shaving in the shower. Rig a mirror and a place to store the razor and shave cream, and have a go. Standing erect, there will be a minimal load on your back, and when you have finished, rinsing has never been easier. (There is now a battery-powered electric razor that operates when the skin is wet, even with shaving cream.)

Self-massage

One of the great benefits of the shower is that you may, while taking it, enjoy a heat treatment and administer a self-massage.

With soap on your hands, your fingers can stroke and knead your shoulders, neck and lower back with ease and effectiveness. As a supplement to your fingers, the soap bar is itself an ideal massage tool.

Precede the massage with a heat treatment. Run the water as reasonably hot as you can bear, with the flow directed onto your back, especially onto the affected area. Not only will the hot water cleanse you, it will draw the tension from the muscles and speed the healing process by increasing the blood flow to the area. (Some elderly people are subject to dizziness in a hot shower. If you are in this age group and in any doubt, take particular care.)

Recovering from a back attack, take a hot shower every day. Take more than one if you feel up to it. Especially, take one before going to sleep. In addition to refreshing you and lowering your tension level, it will contribute to fighting the depression that can so easily descend during the recovery period.

The perils of the bathtub

If you don't have the option of a shower and your back is in a precarious condition, the better part of wisdom is to stay out of the bathtub for the first few days. Make do with a sponge-bath. The average bathtub is booby-trapped in half a dozen ways, and despite the undoubted benefits a warm bath yields, it should be avoided.

However, if you have no shower stall and are the dauntless type and have made up your mind not to be intimidated by the problems, there are measures you can take to minimize the risks.

Most of them have to do with planning ahead. Before you begin, check the following:
- Is there a nonslip surface on the floor of the tub so that you won't take a fall getting in or out?
- If not, is there a rubber mat securely attached to the bathtub surface with multiple suction-cups?
- Is the soap near at hand, where you can reach it without straining?
- Is there a sponge or container handy so that you may rinse your upper arms and shoulders without having to slide down into the water?

- If you have a long-handled brush for scrubbing your
  feet, is it within easy reach?

All these are important details. Once in the tub you
don't want to have to to get out of it for something forgotten or to strain your back by reaching.

Operating the faucets

Bear in mind before beginning to fill the tub that it is a
long way down to the faucets, but a longer way back.
Moreover, the faucets require adjustment to the proper
mix of hot and cold, and accomplishing this can keep you
bent over at an extreme angle for a minute or more. Nor is
it enough at this early stage in your recovery simply to
support your upper body with your free hand on the rim
of the tub. You may get away with it, but it is an unnecessary risk.

Go down to one knee, close enough to the faucets that
you won't have to bend over far. Even then you will want
to support yourself with your free hand because you will
be reaching forward and that greatly increases the load
on your lower back.

A better solution is to have someone run the tub for
you. Indeed, in the earliest stage of your recovery, it is the
better part of wisdom to have someone nearby during
your first attempt to bathe.

Before stepping into the tub, take hold of some support.
It may be the shower rail or a towel rack, even the wall,
but it is important to have a firm hold on something. The
moment one foot is off the floor you are liable to go off
balance, and are therefore at risk. Before you commit
yourself to a support like the towel rack, however, check
that it is secure; you may have to put considerable weight
on it in maintaining your balance. It takes little imagination to envision what could happen if it were suddenly to

give way and you were to fall onto the unforgiving surfaces of the bathroom.

In the tub
Standing in the tub, crouch, place your hands on the rim on both sides and lower your body into the water. Do not extend both legs straight in front of you; doing this will greatly increase the stress on the muscles of the back and could cause a sharp spasm of pain. Take some of the weight by keeping your feet beneath you until your buttocks have touched the bottom of the tub. Then extend your legs, one at a time.

The waters of a warm bath are a gift from the gods. Immersion in moist heat is as relaxing a treatment as sore back muscles can be given. Even though you are in a somewhat cramped situation, the specific gravity of the water will lessen your body weight, and you will find that you are able to lean against the back of the tub, relax and rest with a degree of comfort you may not have felt for days.

Stay put for a few minutes. Enjoy! *But don't remain in this position for long* or you may find it difficult to sit up. It is not unknown for a back-pain victim to relax in the tub too long and then have to call for help to get out.

Having soaped your head and upper body, do not immerse yourself. Wash away the water with squeezings of a sponge or by filling a container and pouring it over yourself. Washing your feet can be a problem because you must lean well forward to do so. A long-handled brush is useful here. If you don't have one, forget your feet.

Getting out of the tub
To get out of the tub, bring one of your feet close to the buttocks, place your hands on the rim of the tub and help

yourself up. Check that the rim and your hands are not slippery with soap; you could slip halfway up and take a bad fall.

Toweling is easy, except for drying your legs and feet. You can go down to one knee and dry one foot at a time or, optionally, put a foot on the toilet seat and bend over until the full weight of your torso is resting on your thigh. With this upper-body support, you will find it is easy to towel your feet.

Do not, however, immediately straighten up. You are bent far over, and the leverage required to raise your torso is extreme. Place a hand (or hands) on your thigh just above the knee and push yourself erect. Then on to the other leg.

As mentioned earlier, always steady yourself and establish your balance before you raise one foot from the floor. Be sure to do this when you go about drying your feet.

10

In the Bathroom

THE DESIGNER WHO FIRST DETERMINED THAT the height of a bathroom-sink countertop should be standardized at approximately 30 to 32 inches should be drummed out of the industrial designers' association on the grounds of inhumanity to sufferers from back pain.

And, as if the low level of the countertop did not present enough problems, the basin over which that individual must bend to perform his or her ablutions is sunk a further 8 to 10 inches.

It is part of an uncoordinated conspiracy against people with back trouble, a global plot that includes the manufacture of overstuffed sofas, angular office chairs, "functional" seating contraptions and geometric designer chairs as resting places for the posteriors of the world — thus, incidentally, contributing to the enrichment of medical doctors, X-ray technicians, osteopaths, chiropractors, acupuncturists, manufacturers of analgesics and an odd-lot of other quirky "specialists."

How can the victims of this conspiracy fight back? Inasmuch as most of us have no option but to use these standardized products, the answer is: only through constant vigilance — and ingenuity.

Fortunately, there are ways to cope.

BEWARE THE BATHROOM

For the person recovering from an acute attack, the bathroom can be the most hazardous room in the house.

One would think the kitchen would be, with its heating elements, electric appliances, scalding liquids and variety of sharp implements, but if you are only recently out of bed, with your muscles weak and your back unstable, the bathroom menaces with even more booby-traps.

We examined in the previous chapter the risks involved in taking a bath or shower — the slippery porcelain areas; the hard, unyielding surfaces if you fall; the contorted confinement of the tub; the foot-tangling bathmat; and the ever-present risk of precipitating a spasm by going off balance.

But the risks go far beyond these. How many back problems have been aggravated by bending low over a sink, by prolonged leaning forward to brush your teeth or shave or put on makeup, not to mention awkward sessions on a toilet seat? Enough to say that the number is beyond reckoning.

But if, as the proverb states, cleanliness is next to godliness, then into the bathroom you must go, even on shaky legs, as soon as you are out of bed and able to manage it.

And it is worth the strain and effort. A session of acute back pain — especially if it is a repeat performance — can create a sense of profound discouragement and bleak depression, even as nothing can contribute more to a buoyancy of spirit and the feeling that you are making progress in your recovery than simply getting yourself squeaky-clean and presentable.

So, don't be deterred by the hazards; they can all be managed.

The bathroom sink
Let's begin with the bathroom sink. It is the first challenge you encounter most mornings, and it can pose real problems.

To begin: the hot and cold faucets require some fine-tuning to achieve the desired water temperature and, with some installations, you may find yourself bent over for the better part of a minute simply to fill the sink.

Coming directly from bed, your back muscles stiff from sleep, it can be a long minute.

There is a simple solution: operate the faucets with one hand. Use your free arm as a prop, resting the hand on the countertop. Or place your hand on the wall or the medicine cabinet in front of you. The outstretched arm will enable you to maintain your back in a straight line as you lean forward. It takes little effort because you are not far off balance. The basin filled, the slightest push will return you to upright.

There is an even simpler option. Rather than face the sink, stand sideways to it. You will discover that you will then be able easily to reach and operate the faucets without bending.

Use either technique any time you need to reach for the soap or the washcloth or to activate the stopper. After a time or two, it will become second nature.

Incidentally, on Day One, position the soap, tooth-paste, toothbrush, washcloth, shaving materials, makeup and other essentials within easy reach on the countertop. There will then be no need to bend over to pick them up.

Standing close

When washing your hands or face, stand as close to the sink as possible. There is usually an undercut at the base of the bathroom cabinet that will allow you to move your feet well forward. So positioned, you automatically reduce the angle required for any leaning you must do.

When bending over the sink to wash and rinse your face, you can greatly reduce the load on your back muscles by the simple expedient of opening the cupboard doors beneath the sink. When you lean forward, you can then freely bend your knees, moving them within the storage space. Crouch as you bend over. This simple action will reduce the angle at which you must bend and will greatly ease the load on your back.

Using the washcloth

Normally, in order to wash your hands, face, ears and neck, you must bend over the sink for prolonged periods. There is a simple alternative: until your back is shipshape again, use a washcloth.

Standing close to the sink, you will find it easy to wet, soap and rinse. If you discover that, while washing, the excess water is dripping onto your body or bathrobe, tie a spare towel loosely around your neck after the fashion of a bib, and that will be taken care of. As well, the towel will be immediately at hand for drying.

The extendable mirror

Shaving or applying makeup poses problems because each requires that you lean close to the mirror to examine the work in progress. And this may necessitate long periods of bending forward.

Again, there is a simple solution: don't move close to the mirror, move the mirror close to you. Buy an extension mirror and mount it on the bathroom wall at eye level. Beyond the advantage of not having to lean forward, the device will enable you to do a better job on your makeup or shaving because one of the mirrors is invariably a magnifier.

If you are a blade-shaver, buy an electric razor — no water, no soap, no rinsing, no dripping, and, even more important, no need to bend over.

Brushing the teeth

Brushing your teeth can prove to be an awkward task; there is invariably some dripping, and normally you must lean forward over the sink.

Again, there is an option.

Keep a spare coffee mug or a ceramic or glass tumbler on the countertop. When brushing your teeth, half fill it with water, and hold it below your chin where any dripping will be caught. When you have finished, place a hand on the wall in front of you, lean forward and expectorate into the sink. Now use the water in the cup for the rinse.

No fuss, no mess and no exacerbation of your back pain.

You can further ease the stress of prolonged standing at the bathroom sink by opening one of the cupboard doors beneath the sink and placing a foot on the raised bottom. This will induce a partial pelvic tilt and will ease the strain on your back. Change feet from time to time, of course.

ON THE THRONE

The waste-elimination functions of the body often grow complicated during a period of extended back pain, which can pose painful and anxiety-inducing problems.

One of the unexpected complications encountered by the first-time victim of a back attack is that, although he or she may be sidelined, life goes on. The normal bodily functions continue. One must eat and drink. One must also eliminate the body's wastes. And the pain of an acute attack or even the discomfort of the recovery period can transform such taken-for-granted activities into worrisome problems.

The digestive system — when the body has been denied normal physical activity, and when it is likely that you have not stuck to your usual pattern of eating — may become sluggish, irregular or dysfunctional. This situation may be intensified by the fact that getting out of bed can often be so fraught with pain and/or trepidation that a trip to the bathroom is postponed or avoided. In such circumstances there are two available options.

Bed pans and potty-chairs

The first is, of course, the bed pan. Unfortunately, during a prolonged back attack, or even when the acute phase has passed, the victim may hover on the edge of further spasms, and a bed pan can pose very real problems.

The old-fashioned bed pan — a bulky, uncomfortable contraption at best — may create more problems than it solves. One must arch the back to get aboard, and that in itself can stimulate sudden jabs of pain.

But adaptation has come, even here. Most drugstores now sell a modern, lightweight version, and if you suffer from frequent or even occasional bouts of back pain, it might be advisable to buy one and keep it available.

It is slim and triangular in profile, the leading edge being no more than one inch deep. The other end is approximately three inches high and includes a handle, making removal from the bed convenient. Uncomfortable though it may be, and intimidating as the prospect may be, it can be inserted beneath the buttocks with a minimum of back arching. It is possible, however, that even this slight elevation of the pelvic area may prove to be too painful. If you have no option, the bed pan can be used as a last resort.

Some victims of acute back pain may be able to get out of bed but be unable to manage the journey to the bathroom. In such a circumstance, a rented potty-chair is the ideal solution. The commode or potty-chair is a collapsible, aluminum-tubing chair of the type commonly described as a "director's chair." Most have a canvas back and, of course, a toilet seat with a removable container beneath.

It is a useful device. It usually rents by the week and is inexpensive. It can be placed immediately beside the bed and has arms on which one can sustain much of one's weight. Moreover, you can get an elevated toilet-seat attachment, making it easier to sit and rise.

You will find a listing in the yellow pages of your telephone book for outlets renting hospital supplies. Most such businesses deliver, or you can have a taxi make a pickup.

The toilet
For the person recovering from a severe back attack, there are few situations more fraught with tension than that interminable wait on the toilet seat — the "consummation devoutly to be wished" that seems momentarily about to be realized, but isn't. And, in the meantime,

twinges, jabs and mini-spasms play about the back like the fitful lightning of a summer storm.

For the victim — especially the larger individual — the average toilet seat can be a place of torment. It is unyielding, uncomfortable and difficult to change position on. The upturned seat cover inclines at an awkward angle and makes an uncomfortable backrest. Worse, it provides poor support for the lower back. Little wonder the victim of a back attack can come to dread nature's command.

Again, fortunately, much can be done about it.

To begin, roll a small bath towel into a cylinder and position it in the declivity at the bottom of the backrest. It will add a degree of comfort, support your lower back and help you to establish and sustain the pelvic tilt.

Place a telephone book on the floor in front of the toilet bowl. Use it as a place to put your feet, thus elevating your knees higher than your hips. If your city directory is thin, improvise with an upside-down desk drawer or something similar.

Don't sit rigid and unmoving; vary your position from time to time by leaning forward to rest your hands or elbows on your thighs. After doing so, however, exercise caution in straightening up. Take it slowly, and assist the back muscles by pushing on your thighs.

Prepare a number of sheets of toilet tissue in advance so that you do not have to twist about reaching for them. A convenient solution is to place a box of "man-size" tissues near to hand. Each can be folded two or three times in one use, thus minimizing the reaching and twisting normally involved.

Irregularity and laxatives

Confinement to bed, decreased physical activity, altered eating habits and even the constriction of the colon induced by tension may soon lead to a sluggish bowel.

There would seem to be a correlation between low back pain and constipation. Men especially may discover that the normal urination and evacuation signals become untrustworthy and that either or both may signal false alarms. (Incidentally, keep a urinal bottle on the night table by the bed; it will save you many trips to the bathroom.)

The common problem is, of course, constipation. A buildup of fecal matter in the colon can itself intensify your low back pain and, if it continues unremedied for an extended period of time, can complicate your recuperation.

In such circumstances there will be a tendency to strain, and this should be avoided. If no progress is made after a few minutes, get up and move around. And because being immobilized can exacerbate the stiffness and soreness of your back, use self-massage frequently.

Remedies

Constipation is a frequent problem for many as a result of unwise eating habits — mostly the ingestion of refined foods containing little fiber or roughage. As a consequence, irregularity in emptying the bowels and a subsequent dependency on laxatives develops. Unfortunately, the laxative cure often worsens the problem. With little bulk in the fecal matter, the normal peristaltic action (successive waves of contraction moving along the intestine) cannot function effectively. Consequently, more laxatives are taken, the cycle is intensified and the condition becomes chronic.

How should the sufferer from back pain deal with the problem?

Change your diet: eat salads and fresh fruits, and cereals noted for their roughage content. Ideally, the cereal should contain large proportions of seeds, whole grains and chopped nuts along with dried fruits. A variety of such cereals is available everywhere.

If a supplement becomes necessary, most health-food stores and many chiropractors recommend laxatives made from a blend of herbal fiber. They are effective for some but can have adverse effects for others. Regardless, the taking of regular doses of *any* laxative is a bad habit to get started on. The pleasant, old-fashioned remedy of eating a few prunes daily (three to five, and only as required) seems an ideal solution.

If three full days have passed without an evacuation, have a word with your doctor.

11

Why Your Back Hurts

MANY SUFFERERS FROM BACK PAIN BECOME THE captives of their fear. Their lives are dogged by a constant anxiety, an overriding concern that one wrong move may "put their back out" again and incapacitate them, perhaps threaten their livelihood, their physical activities, even their lifestyle.

We have an abnormal concern for the back, an almost atavistic fear. It can be seen even in childish concerns about the most dread afflictions: "Step on a crack; break your mother's back," we chant as children. We talk about "breaking the back" of a tough job. We feel a special pity for the paralytic confined to a wheelchair, lower limbs wasted and useless. We observe with a macabre fascination as one of the great cats leaps onto the back of its prey and kills it by severing the spinal cord. We watch a dog catch a rat and dispatch it with a vigorous shaking, breaking its back.

There is a tendency to think of the back as a place of special vulnerability, as the weak link in our physiology — "After all, we weren't *supposed* to walk on two feet." Perhaps the concern is derivative of a race memory. Among our forbears, the man who injured his back would become a liability, someone who stayed at home with the women and children while the men of the tribe went off to hunt.

WORRYING ABOUT YOUR BACK

Contrary to common belief, the human back is not a weak link in our physical makeup. Nor is "a bad back," as we tend to call it, a mysterious, malevolent enemy lying in wait, ready to sideline you for days or weeks if you make a careless move, causing you pain, limiting your activity and robbing you of much that is enjoyable in life.

Indeed, an undue concern about the back is itself a harmful thing, as worry and tension are among the major causes of back problems. People who suffer a back attack and brood about a recurrence make the recurrence more likely. Some live under the shadow of the initial affliction and become self-made invalids. You may recognize some of the signs; you may even display some of them:

- They frequent medical offices and repeatedly change doctors.
- They become chronic complainers, describing to anyone who will listen the specifics of "my back problem."
- They walk with cautious steps, often with a hand pressed to the small of the back.
- They suffer frequent relapses that put them in bed for a few hours or a few days.
- They vow often to undertake a regimen of exercise (and do sometimes begin), only to abandon it after a few days or weeks.

- They have been treated by GPS, chiropractors, osteopaths, masseurs, acupuncturists, hypnotherapists and yoga masters, about whom they, at first, enthuse but soon abandon.
- They have read all the books on back problems available in the Health section of the local bookstore or library.

The fear of acute back pain is understandable — the suffering *can* be great and the recovery period can be incapacitating — but, more often than not, the reaction is disproportionate to the actual problem.

Granted, the pain may be considerable, but if there is no physiological abnormality (and this is true in at least 90 percent of cases), while the attack may be distressing, even temporarily incapacitating, it will, in all probability, be short-lived and will surely pass with time.

More important: something *can* be done about it.

Unfortunately, undue apprehension and the consequent "cautionary tension," as we think of it, are among the major causes of chronic back pain. Continue to fret about the possibility of a recurrence and that very concern may contribute to further attacks.

AN ENGINEERING MARVEL
It may help to know something about the construction and functioning of your back. Many a bogeyman in the closet disappears when the light is turned on.

The human body is a complex and awe-inspiring organism. In prescientific times, philosophers marveled at its mysteries and poets rhapsodized about its beauty. And little wonder — it is a marvel of engineering and a "mechanism" of incredible versatility.

We understand it better than our forbears did, and most of its mysteries have become familiar territory to the contemporary medical practitioner. Granted that, as is true of every complex part of the body, there are mysteries yet unexplored, the human spine is an essentially simple mechanism.

The spine is the infrastructure on which the upper body is supported. It comprises thirty-three or thirty-four bones, all of them bound together and activated by muscles, ligaments and tendons. The ligaments join bones to other bones, or to cartilage in the joint areas. The tendons serve to connect muscle to bone and the muscles provide the support and the power. Movement is accomplished when the muscles contract and/or relax.

Despite this essential simplicity, the variety of movement, the versatility and the power of the body is astonishing. We marvel at the fluid grace of the ballet dancer and watch open-mouthed as the Olympic heavyweight lofts three times his own weight above his head. It is the more astonishing when we realize that all of this power and versatility — and much more — stems from the ability of each muscle to do the one thing it is designed to do: to contract!

The muscles are highly specialized bands of tissues consisting mostly of elongated cells. When stimulated by the nervous system, the muscles contract and thus pull on or hold stationary the related bones. As mentioned above, this is all a muscle can do — contract. Happily, the end result of this essentially simple process is movement almost without limit.

And all of it is anchored on and proceeds from the spine.

The spine
The most complex arrangement of bones in your body is found in the spine. The very fact that it is vertical makes us unique among mammals. It is a marvel of versatility, having the capacity to move and twist and bend in almost

any direction. The most complex mechanisms devised by the combined skills of our best technicians to imitate its actions are crude and cumbersome by comparison.

As mentioned above, the spine is formed by thirty-three or thirty-four vertebrae, divided into five principal sections.

At the top are the seven so-called *cervical* vertebrae forming the neck, the first two being attached to and supporting the skull. The cervical vertebrae are extraordinarily flexible, more so than any other part of the spine.

Next come the twelve *thoracic* vertebrae, each attached to individual ribs and serving to contain and protect such vital organs as the heart, the lungs and the liver. Because each of the thoracic vertebrae is attached to a pair of ribs (and the ribs in pairs to each other), it is capable of relatively little movement.

Below this are the five *lumbar* vertebrae. They form what is commonly called the low back, the locus of most back problems. The lumbar area is capable of considerable movement, being able to flex and bend and rotate, within limits, in all directions.

Below these are the five *sacral* vertebrae, the so-called tailbone. They are fused to each other and to the hip bones, or pelvis, and act to support and protect the bladder and the reproductive organs, and to provide, among other things, a solid area of connection and leverage for the thigh bones and muscles.

At the base of the spine are the three to five (some people have three, others five, most four) fused segments called the coccyx.

Standing tall

When our forbears changed their habitat from the trees to the ground and found it advantageous to stand on their hind legs, this eventually effected major changes in the body's center of gravity and brought about a radical difference from most other mammals in the functioning of the spine. To sustain the body in this unnatural upright position required changes in the shape of the spine and altered the operation of various muscles.

The forces of gravity working on the human body and on the body of a quadruped are radically different. In four-footed mammals, the center of gravity lies normally between the front and rear legs. The spine is supported at both ends, and the gravitational pull is absorbed from one end to the other. In a human, standing erect, the gravitational forces are all exerted vertically, and any deviation from vertical requires a balancing act that affects, to various degrees, virtually every muscle of the body.

There is a difference also in the way we and the quadrupeds absorb impact, and therein lies many of our problems. When your cat, for instance, leaps from a height, the impact is distributed horizontally, the force being taken on the front paws and transferred though the bowed spine, all the way to the rear. When a human leaps to the ground, the impact is absorbed vertically. Much of it is lessened by a flexing of the leg muscles, but the remainder must be absorbed by the spinal column or the jolt delivered to the torso, neck and and head could be severe. Happily, the shape of the spine — a flexible, flattened S-curve — provides a shock-absorber and offers the required resilience.

The vertebrae
The vertebrae differ from each other in size and function. Most of them consist of drum-shaped bones from which seven projections extend. Toward the back of each vertebra is a vertical hole that, when the vertebrae are

stacked on top of each other, forms a canal that runs the length of the spine. This canal encloses and protects the spinal cord, that complex collection of nerve fibres that connects the brain to the various parts of the body. Bundles of "nerve-roots," as they are called, branch out to different parts of the body through small openings between the vertebrae and, basically, control the movement and transmit sensory information to and from that area and the brain.

One of the seven bony protrusions on each vertebra extends straight back and is the part of the spine you can feel when you run your fingers down your back. Two of the protrusions extend sideways and are the means by which the back muscles attach to and move the spine. The other four (two pairs) are called "facets" and make the spine the firm but flexible unit it is by intersecting with matching facets on the vertebrae immediately above and below. Each is capped with smooth, white cartilage (think of the "knuckle-bone" on a chicken drumstick) so that, where they intersect with other facets, there is virtually no friction. To keep them interfaced but free to move, they are enclosed in a tough, fibrous casing. And lest you think they are insecurely joined, you can more easily dislocate your shoulder than a facet joint.

The vertebrae are further supported by powerful muscles running along both sides of the spine, from top to bottom.

The discs
The individual vertebrae are separated by tough but malleable cushioning units called discs. Their function is to maintain a separation of the vertebrae, to help absorb shocks and to permit flexibility.

The exterior walls of a disc are made of tough, interwoven fibrous cartilage. (They have been aptly likened to the walls of radial tires.) The discs are, themselves, filled with a thick gelatinous substance. This substance, which is 90 percent water in a newborn, slowly loses some of its liquid content over the years, and this dehydration slightly diminishes the thickness of the disc, sometimes causing the facet joints to become misaligned, producing what is commonly described as joint pain.

It is interesting that, under the pressure of your body weight, a disc may lose as much as 10 percent of its thickness through the day; that is the reason you are taller in the morning than at night (as much as an inch). Normal thickness is regained as you sleep. This variability was dramatically illustrated when men began to travel in space, where the gravitational pull is negligible. It was discovered during their first extended sojourn that the astronauts' height increased, making their precisely tailored spacesuits uncomfortable.

As the space between the vertebrae lessens with the years, pressures may begin to impinge on the nerve roots where they pass from the spinal canal to various parts of the body. This may occasionally or chronically cause pain or tingling or numbness in areas that may be distant from and seem unrelated to the back. These "phantom" pains can usually be tracked to their source only by a doctor.

YOUR SORE BACK: A SPRAINED MUSCLE
What happens when you injure your back? Setting aside disease, structural abnormality and a ruptured disc, your sore back is not much different in kind from a sprained muscle.

You may, at some time in your life, have sprained an ankle. What happened when you did? The joint where two or more bones intersected was forced too far out of line, and some of the related muscles were stressed beyond their limits and tore. They didn't tear loose but, depending on the seriousness of the injury, some of the muscle fibers ruptured. As a result, you couldn't put your body weight on the ankle without suffering pain.

Generally, when you "pull a muscle in your back," the same sort of thing happens. Stressed beyond its capacity, the ruptured muscle signals the injury via the nervous system to the brain, and you feel pain.

Much of the pain may stem, however, from a secondary cause. Often, when muscles controlled by the brain are injured (as, for instance, when you strain your back while lifting) the surrounding muscles, controlled by the autonomic nervous system, try to minimize the damage by going rigid.

As we have seen, this automatic protective reaction may produce muscle spasm, and inasmuch as muscles in spasm do not heed messages from the brain telling them to relax, they can produce the prolonged and excruciating suffering often experienced by the victim of an acute back attack.

Unfortunately, the pain produced by muscle spasm may continue for an indefinite period, ranging from a few seconds to a few hours, or even longer. When the spasm eases and nature begins the healing process, the originally damaged muscles become the principal concern. As a result of the initial sprain, inflammation and swelling occur, and this damage must go through the healing process.

The extent of the damage determines, in large part, the time required for your recovery.

12

Bending and Lifting

IT IS PROBABLE THAT MORE BACK INJURIES ARE caused by lifting and twisting than in any other way.

If you want to avoid such problems, you need to know something about the fundamentals of human body-mechanics — specifically, how your body functions when you stand, walk, run, sit, bend, kneel, squat or lift.

The human body is a magnificent mechanism, but it is vulnerable. Disregard its limitations and you may sprain a muscle, damage tissue, even permanently incapacitate yourself.

And few parts of the human anatomy are more subject to frequent injury than is the back.

From that moment in early childhood when you did that uniquely human thing, stand erect, you have been engaged in an unremitting war with gravity. Our physical uniqueness among mammals derives from the muscles of the lower back and those that coordinate with them. It is their ability to "lever" the upper part of the body erect and sustain it in that position that makes us different from other creatures and provides many of the advantages that enabled our forbears to become the dominant species on earth.

Viewed simply, in engineering terms, straightening up after bending over is an extraordinary achievement. To accomplish it, the muscles of the back and stomach must lever half the body's weight from horizontal to vertical without external assistance.

Standing upright is "unnatural," and returning to vertical after bending over can make great demands on the lower back. That we can accomplish this — and normally do it with ease — becomes even more remarkable when you realize that we frequently do so while lifting heavy objects.

BENDING OVER

What keeps us from falling forward when we bend over?

When maintaining a stable upright stance, we do so by positioning half our body weight on each side of an imaginary vertical line running from the ear to the ankle.

However, innumerable times each day we must depart from the vertical — to tie a shoelace, to pick up the morning newspaper, to retrieve something we have dropped or simply to pat the dog — and this must be done without either falling forward or straining the back muscles when we straighten up.

But we go far beyond this: we frequently lift heavy loads and engage in what is commonly described as "backbreaking labor."

To avoid damaging the back, some understanding of what your body can and cannot do is essential. Knowing your capabilities and your limitations helps because it enables you to avoid unwise or precipitate actions and thus reduces the possibility of injury.

There are four ways to bend over without going off balance. In each of them you so rearrange the principal segments of your body that exactly half your weight is positioned on each side of an imaginary vertical line.

This sounds complex but it isn't — we do it every day, and do it without conscious thought. The four ways are:

1. by moving the upper body forward and the posterior back,
2. by bending at the knees and hips,
3. by going to one knee, and
4. by squatting.

Bending over without bending your knees is the most stressful of the four postures.

Such an action makes great demands on the muscles of the low back. And, if while bending forward, you pick up something heavy — thus adding to the load on your lower back — you not only stretch the muscles to their limit, you require them, in that stressed condition, to exert maximum leverage to return the torso to upright.

This poses no great problem for the young or the fit, but it can be risky for the average adult and downright dangerous for the man or woman out of shape.

You have seen children or dancers or gymnasts bend far over, even put their head between their legs. Require the sedentary middle-age man to do the same and he will end up on the floor in pain.

Therefore, it is the better part of wisdom never to bend over with your knees locked.

Few actions can subject the back muscles to a greater load. And, if you have bent over to lift a heavy object from the floor, you are not only requiring your back muscles to stretch to the limit, you are calling on them to exert maximum leverage in returning to upright.

Fix the rule in your subconscious: *never bend over without bending your knees.* It can save you much grief.

GETTING CLOSE TO THE FLOOR
Bending the knees while bending over automatically reduces the risks involved for a number of reasons.

By bending your knees, you reduce your height. Consequently, you no longer need to angle your back so far forward in reaching to the floor. And because you have lessened the angle at which your back is bent, you have reduced the load on the low back when you straighten up.

You have a second option: *you can go to one knee.*

In doing this, you immediately solve two problems: you further reduce your height and therefore no longer need to bend your back at an extreme angle when you reach down. In going to one knee, you so arrange your body weight that it remains in equilibrium. Moreover, you are now stabilized at three points rather than two: the knee, the extended front foot and the toe of the rear foot. There is a further benefit: if you must remain bent over for a prolonged period, you can lessen the load on your back by resting a forearm on your thigh.

There is a third option, which may, at times, be even more advantageous: *you can squat.*

In doing so, you again reduce your height and thus make it easy to reach the floor without bending far forward. As well, you make heavy lifting easier. You are able to bring the load closer to your body and can make the lift with your back straight, the heavy work being assigned to the thighs.

Squatting has one disadvantage, however; it is not as

stable a posture as going to one knee where you have three points of contact with the floor. As a consequence, you are more subject to going off balance.

It is a good rule to squat only when there is a third point of support within reach: a wall, a chair, a table or whatever.

STRAIGHTENING UP

Contrary to what is widely believed, you do not injure your back by bending over. It is injured when, *having bent over, you begin to straighten up.*

You may have heard a victim of back pain say, "It's murder when I bend over." This is incorrect. It does not hurt when you bend over; it hurts the moment you begin to straighten up. As you lean forward, the muscles of the low back merely control the rapidity and direction of the upper body's descent. The injury takes place when the muscles of the low back are called upon to maintain the bent-over posture or to return the torso to upright.

Paradoxically, there is great comfort in knowing this.

The knowledge that bending forward will not, of itself, hurt you can greatly lessen the fear of a back attack. You will know that, in any normal circumstance, you may bend over without risk. And you will know also that you may be at risk, at imminent risk, *the moment when, having arrested the forward movement, you begin to reverse it.*

Knowing when and why you are at risk enables you to guard against injury. Rather than straighten up thoughtlessly, the Automatic Response System (see the final chapter) in your subconscious will automatically slow the return to upright. Or it will lessen the load on the back muscles by cueing you to place your hands on your thighs or on a nearby object in order to assist.

These facts in mind, establish firmly in your subconscious the following rules for guarding against overstressing the back muscles:

FOUR RULES FOR BENDING OVER

1. *Never bend forward with your knees locked.* When the knees are locked, the pelvis remains high, requiring you to bend down farther than you would if your knees were bent.
2. *The farther you bend over, the more your knees must be flexed.* This flexing lowers the upper part of your body and brings you closer to the floor. As well, it transfers some of the load to the buttocks and hamstring muscles, thus reducing the demand on your back.
3. *Having bent over for an extended time, do not straighten up suddenly.* The muscles will be fatigued and may lack resiliency. First, reduce the load on your back by placing your hands on your thighs. Then straighten up — but slowly.
4. *If you feel your back muscles at risk, "walk" your hands up your thighs until you are erect.* Optionally, place a hand on to a nearby stable object and assist your return to vertical.

THREE RULES FOR LIFTING

As should be obvious: if you pick up a heavy object while bent over incorrectly, "Somethin's gotta give." That "something" is, of course, one or more of the muscles of your lower back.

There are three basic rules for lifting:
1. Keep the object to be lifted close to your body.
2. Lift with your thighs, not with your arms and back.
3. Never turn while lifting without first shifting your lead foot in the direction you wish to go.

Dr. Hamilton Hall, the Canadian back specialist, summarized Rule One in a memorable phrase: "Never take out the garbage in your Sunday suit." He then improved on that with the question: "Have you hugged your garbage can today?"

Obviously, if you are wearing good clothes you will tend to hold lifted objects away from the body, thus greatly increasing the leverage factor on the back. Doing so can sprain a muscle or even inflict damage on one or more of your facet joints. The damage may not be severe and will usually heal, but the after-effects can linger in a soreness or susceptibility to further strains that can dog your days.

Next time you must lift a heavy object remember these facts:

- Raised from the floor with the knees locked, a load weighing 20 pounds can exert 200 pounds of pressure on the lower back.
- Raised at arm's length, away from the body, *it can exert an additional 200 pounds.*

When you have a load to lift, keep your back relatively erect and either go to one knee or squat. You may have observed that Olympic weight lifters use both of these techniques in their routines. As noted earlier — the disadvantage of the squat is that you can easily go off balance. The reason is obvious: to begin the lift while squatting, you must lean forward — and this is especially true if the load is wider than can comfortably be brought close with your knees spread.

Usually, it is better to use a diagonal stance when squatting — one foot in front of the other, both knees bent. Better still, go to one knee. This stance provides better stability and enables you to bring the load close to your body while maintaining your back in a relatively erect position.

Lifting is a situation in which you benefit from having learned the pelvic tilt. Move close to the load and tuck in your pelvis just before you make the lift. It will minimize the stress on your lower back. You will make the lift with less jeopardy if your stomach muscles are in good shape. *Fit stomach muscles are absolutely essential to heavy lifting.*

AVOIDING TROUBLE
If you have a heavy object to lift and are subject to recurring back problems, forget all the counsel offered above and get help. Optionally, divide the load into two. Or use a lifting device. It is foolish, and dangerous, to struggle with a heavy load if there is an available option.

There are, of course, any number of objects to be lifted in the course of the average day, ranging from an infant in its playpen, to a sack of groceries, to a shovel full of snow.

Men whose children have grown to adulthood and are beginning to raise their own families find themselves surprised at how heavy babies are. Carrying them, one is reminded of a line of Shakespeare's: "this too too solid flesh." However, it is commonplace for young mothers to bend to the floor or into playpens to pick up infants or toddlers — and to reach far forward to do it. Little wonder so many women of childrearing age are subject to back pain.

Again, the mandatory rule applies: *bend the knees and bring the object close.*

TWISTING WHILE LIFTING
The risk of serious damage to the back occurs when you turn while lifting. Not only is there the possibility of muscle injury, there is the risk of doing damage to the facet joints or to the discs, those flexible "joints" between the vertebrae.

The vertebrae of the low back are relatively large (as compared, for instance, to those in the neck) and, compared to those in the neck, are much less flexible. You can rotate your neck almost 100 degrees. The lumbar discs cannot be turned nearly so much — their principal function being to provide load-bearing strength and stability. Forcing them to rotate while under pressure can put great stress on both the facet joints and the discs. You are particularly likely to damage the discs if you are approaching or have passed your middle years and the discs have begun the slow dehydration that comes with aging.

Undoing the twist

How can you avoid the risk? *By pivoting rather than twisting.*

The difference is this:

- When you twist, you turn the torso without moving your feet, and the farther you turn the greater the amount of torque imposed on the spine.
- When you pivot, you first turn your feet in the direction you intend to move so that your feet (or at least the lead foot) are maintained in line with your shoulders and hips.

Keep this at the forefront of your mind when you are shoveling snow, spading in the garden or repetitively moving a number of objects. There is a particular risk attached to repeatedly filling a shovel and then, without shifting your feet, turning to pitch it aside.

And this is particularly true if your muscles are cold.

Turning while bending over

One of the easiest ways to "put your back out" is to twist while bent over.

It is easy to understand why: with the muscles drawn taut to sustain the back in the bent-over position, you turn. Suddenly, the load is slackened on the muscles of one side of the back and intensified on the other, in effect, doubling the load on those muscles.

The precaution is simple: *avoid turning while bent over*.

If the move is necessary or unavoidable, first move your feet in the desired direction, making certain that your knees are bent as you start the turn, then begin it with the hips rather than with the shoulders.

LOWERING A LOAD

Loads that are picked up must be set down, and both actions can create dicey situations. Indeed, putting the load down may prove the more difficult, simply because your muscles have fatigued.

Because you are about to have done with that pesky box or carton or whatever, there is a tendency to grow careless in putting it down. The knees are not bent and the in-close lifting position is momentarily forgotten.

Use the same care in setting down a load as in lifting it. Here is a useful hint: If the object is not fragile, lower it part way and then drop it. You will thus avoid entering the danger zone.

Yogi Berra said of a baseball game, "The game isn't over 'til it's over." The same is true of lifting and carrying.

13

Sitting

A SENIOR EXECUTIVE IN A LARGE CORPORATION, A man whose life has more than its share of tension, was talking about his battle with low-back pain.

"I can't figure it out," he was saying. "I don't do any lifting. I'm not into strenuous sports. At work I spend most of my day seated at my desk. I spend my evenings relaxing in the most comfortable chair I can find. And yet I have constant trouble with my back. It doesn't make sense."

It does, of course. Unfortunately, he was under the impression — as many are — that sitting is easy on the back.

But as the song in *Porgy and Bess* says: "It ain't necessarily so."

STRESS WHILE SEATED

Ours is a sedentary age. While it is true that there are more men and women jogging or working out than at any time in recent history, it seems likely that our generation does more sitting than any that has preceded it.

- We sit at a desk at our place of work.
- We sit on assembly-lines.
- We sit in front of computer screens and typewriters.
- We sit to talk on the telephone.
- We sit at counters or tables to lunch.
- We sit (wishful thinking!) on buses and subways.
- We sit for extended periods on planes and trains.
- We sit in traffic — sometimes for hours.
- We sit in restaurants and perch on bar-stools.
- We sit at the movies and at sports events.
- We sit before television screens through the evening.
- We sit to read a newspaper or a book.

It would seem reasonable to assume that sitting would be restful for the back — after all, do we not sit down to rest? Unfortunately, this assumption may be false. In certain circumstances, in fact, the opposite may be true.

In the 1970s, the definitive study on posture and its relation to stresses on the back was done in Goteborg, Sweden. The testing measured the relative pressures on the lumbar discs (the lower back) produced by the most common attitudes of the body, ranging from lying flat on your back to standing bent over. The results were surprising, and in many cases contradicted the conventional wisdom.

Most surprising was the finding that *the load on the low back is greater when you are seated and leaning forward than it is when you are standing and bent over*.

There was another unexpected finding: namely, that the load on the discs of your low back while slumped in an easy chair reading or watching television may be greater than when you are standing.

This being so, it might be wise to review your sitting habits and the design of the chairs you sit in — at work and in the comfort of your living room.

THE OFFICE CHAIR (MANAGERIAL)

It may be assumed that, because the type of chair provided for senior personnel and executives is usually larger and more expensive than those provided for other members of the staff, it will be designed with an understanding of the body's mechanics and be easy on the back. This may not be so.

The chair may be impressive, leather-upholstered, segmented and subject to being adjusted to half a dozen positions, and yet be hard on the back. And don't make the mistake of assuming that because the chair is costly it is therefore utilitarian.

Much of the work done by managerial types calls for two basic seated positions: leaning forward to do desk work and tilting back for conferences and conversation.

Frequently, the chair that is comfortable for relaxing in is ill-suited for desk work. Sitting forward for extended periods on the edge of a chair that has a kind of bucket seat can be exceedingly stressful. The seat will tend to tilt you backward and will force you to compensate by straining forward. Few things can be more fatiguing over the period of a day. Leaning forward while seated is stressful on the back; straining forward is worse.

The problem can sometimes be corrected by altering the plane of the seat surface or by using a shallow cushion. Failing that, get another chair, even if it has no fancy adjustments and doesn't match the decor of your office.

And look critically at other aspects of the chair. If the seat is too high or too low, it will, in the first instance, require you to strain far forward or, in the second, will put undue pressure on the lumbar discs and the muscles of the low back.

As with any chair used while working, yours should be at a height that will enable you to sit with your feet comfortably and firmly on the floor. Nor should it be so deep that you have either to shift forward or to bend far over to work on the surface of your desk.

If no other solution is available, get a small firm cushion and place it behind your back.

If you are in your chair most of the day it is good practice to change your posture frequently. Pull out a desk drawer and prop a foot on it. Cross your legs once in a while — but not always the same leg. Get a clipboard and let it substitute from time to time for the top of your desk. Lean back while you make notes or draft a lengthy document. There is a clipboard now available in back-stores that has a pillow of sorts attached to the bottom. When placed on your lap, it raises the surface to a comfortable height and is stable for working on, even with your knees crossed.

Other possibilities:

- If you have been working at your desk for a prolonged period, tilt the chair back, put your feet on the desk and use the moment for relaxation and thought.
- Take most telephone calls standing up. Or perch briefly on a corner of your desk.
- Get out of your chair from time to time. Go for a brief stroll about the office. If your office isn't that spacious, at least circle your desk.

- Working on a knotty problem, stand at the window and look out, unfocused, at the view.
- Place your hands on the small of the back and give yourself a brief massage. It relaxes the muscles and stimulates the blood flow in the area.
- Roll up a small towel and place it behind your lower back. You'll soon discover where to position it. Back stores sell small flexible supports for the purpose.
- Get a secondary stand-up desk; ideally one with a foot bar. This allows you to stand with the knee flexed, thus reducing tension on the low back.

Maintaining your chair tilted backward during conversation or prolonged telephone calls can provide a useful change of posture. Persisted in for long periods, however, it can play havoc with the neck and shoulder muscles. It requires the neck to be bent forward while maintaining eye contact with associates, which can lead to back fatigue or, more likely, to stiffness in the neck.

In normal sitting, don't slump. Rather, shove your tailbone into the back of the chair. This will provide support for your lower back. If you are made uncomfortable by this position, it is probable that your chair, for all its impressiveness, is orthopedically unsound.

If you have been sitting for an extended period, take particular care when getting to your feet. Push the chair back, place your hands on the arms and slide your buttocks to the edge of the seat. Bring your feet beneath you and, with a slight assist from your arms if needed, rise straight up.

In rising from a chair, the rule is: *get your back straight, then stand*. You will find that the sequence will become second nature and you will do it without conscious thought.

THE OFFICE CHAIR (SECRETARIAL)

If your work requires you to sit for hours before a computer or a typewriter, you will want to make doubly certain that your chair gives your back adequate support.

Most secretarial chairs have mechanisms that can be adjusted. Raise or lower the back section so that it provides support for the small of your back. If it isn't adjustable, use a small cushion.

The seat should be set at a height that enables you to rest your feet flat on the floor. And it should be deep enough that it supports most of the length of your thighs, thus distributing the weight of the upper body. If you are subject to back pain, you may find it useful to put a low footstool or a spare telephone book beneath the desk so that you can prop your feet on it, thus achieving a partial pelvic tilt. Ideally, the knees will be slightly higher than your hips.

While you're at it, check the distance of your chair from the desk. If you are requiring yourself habitually to lean forward while working, you are asking for trouble.

But don't make the mistake of slavishly maintaining one position; vary it. And get up for a few minutes every once in a while. It improves the circulation and can do much to relax the muscles of your back, shoulders and neck.

Make certain that the computer screen you look at all day is slightly below eye level and directly in front of you. (This should also be true of your dictation notebook if you work at a typewriter.) You can determine the angle simply by noting the position of your head when you look at the screen. Your head should be as it would be when you are standing and engaged in normal conversation with others of your height. Constantly looking down, or up, or off to one side while working will create sore neck and shoulder muscles, and may even aggravate a vulnerable back.

If you wear bifocals, get a pair of single-lens glasses for work. Bifocals are useful in many ways but they often require you to tilt your head back, which can play havoc with your neck.

THE OFFICE CHAIR (STAFF)

If at work you sit on a standard straight-back chair, follow the general suggestions made about back support and the avoidance of muscle fatigue noted above — with these additions:

If your chair doesn't have arms, try to wangle one that does. Not only will the arms help to relieve some of the weight of your upper body on the lower back but they will make getting into and out of the chair easier.

It may be that your work requires you to sit on a stool or a high-standing chair. This can become an exceedingly uncomfortable perch as the day wears on. As a matter of fact, it would be difficult to design a more effective instrument of torture than a backless high stool.

If it (or any other chair) becomes intolerable, have a word with your company superior. Draw it to his or her attention that you suffer from a bad back and that the seating provided is hindering you from doing your work well. If you explain the problem in a tone that is neither complaining nor challenging, it will probably be given consideration. Any sensibly run company knows that productivity is much affected by the circumstances of the workplace and will look at your problem with some sympathy.

If your appeal is dismissed or disregarded, you will be left with only two options: to quit or to do what can be done to adapt.

The best solution is to change position as often as is feasible. Perch with your buttocks smack-dab on the top of the stool and, if possible, place your heels on one of the rungs. Try, if possible, to get your knees slightly higher than the top of the stool. There are usually rungs at two levels. Place one foot on each level and change about when the need is felt.

Sit with one side of your buttocks on the stool and one foot on the floor. This position will distort the line of your spine, of course, and will be tiring if sustained, so change about frequently.

From time to time, get off the stool and stand as you work. The reason for all this changing about is to keep particular muscles from being under sustained strain. If you distribute the load to a variety of muscles by changing your posture, the fatigue factor will be lessened.

If yours is a high-standing chair with a back, you will be better off, but only slightly. In addition to the changes in posture listed above, you will also be able to position a cushion behind your back, which may provide some support.

If your company is indifferent to your sitting problems, it will help your spirits, if not your back, if you buy a stuffed animal, name it after your boss and stick pins in it nightly.

SITTING ABOUT AT HOME

One of the many illusions held about chairs is the widely held one that, because a chair is overstuffed or down-filled, it is good for the back.

A few years back there was a vogue for those squat, simulated leather hassocks filled with (so it was said) beans. It was commonly believed that these ugly, misbegotten pieces of furniture were ideal for the sufferer from back discomfort.

"Why not?" their advocates argued. The declivity into which you sank could be kneaded, punched and molded to conform to your posterior and would therefore provide the ideal, individualized back support.

One user vividly remembers finding himself almost inextricably trapped in a semi-recumbent sprawl in one of these glorified beanbags, unable either to move or to struggle up from it without help.

Few pieces of "furniture" have been so ill-designed for their purpose. After you had finished your burrowing and had deposited your buttocks in the cavity, you found yourself leaning back awkwardly with the mid and upper parts of your torso unsupported and your neck under strain to avoid staring at the ceiling.

The overupholstered easy-chair ("Just let yourself sink back into it") can be deceptive. You sink into it, and in the first flush of downy suspension don't realize that two deleterious things are happening: first, your buttocks and upper back are being supported but the small of your back is not; and, second, in order to engage in conversation, read or watch the television screen, your head must be craned forward.

In the first instance your lower back is going to tire, and in the second you are going to get a pain in the neck.

Any time you plan to sit for a protracted period (as, for instance, when reading a book or watching TV), make certain that your lower back is supported and that, rather than semi-reclining, you are sitting.

In any case, no matter how comfortable you may be, don't settle in for the evening. Get up every so often and move about. Change your position frequently. Stretch your muscles and keep the blood moving. You'll be better for it.

If you are recovering from the acute phase of a back attack and have settled down before the television set, take particular care to change position from time to time. You may want to rest your back for a few minutes by lying on the carpet. Don't, however, make the mistake of doing so and then tilting your head forward to see the screen. Make do with the audio portion and an occasional peek at the action.

If you are seated fairly upright, put your feet on a low footstool or some makeshift device so that your knees are above your hips. And cross your legs from time to time (but not for prolonged periods); it alters the areas of stress. If you are limber, you may even want to crouch for a few minutes in a corner, steadied by the intersecting walls. Don't stay there too long, though; you may find that you can't get up unassisted.

SPECIALIZED CHAIRS
If your back is a chronic problem, you should investigate the specialized back chairs on the market.

Sitting before the computer screen for hours was a major problem for one of the authors of this book until he purchased a special contour chair. It was fairly expensive but worth every penny of it. It is now possible to work for long hours without back discomfort. The chair can be raised, lowered and tilted, and it has a contoured form that matches the "S" curve of the back. As well, it has arms at the right height, it swivels and it rests on five legs for stability.

There is a revolutionary new chair on the market called the Balans chair. The design originated in Denmark, and it is unlike any chair you have ever seen. The unorthodox seat tilts you forward so that your thighs angle downward and your knees rest on a padded support. The position requires you to maintain the spine in an upright position with a normal curve in the lumbar region. The usual pressures on the disks in that area are eased by the transfer of much of your upper-body weight to the knees. Some find it a godsend; others can't endure it for five minutes. If you have bad knees or are overweight, forget it. Otherwise, you may want to check it out at a back store.

Having referred to most of the new therapeutic chairs, let us remind you of one of the most traditional, the rocker. Although used for centuries as a means of relaxation, particularly by the elderly, it regained popularity in the 1960s when the then president of the United States, John F. Kennedy, injured his back while planting a memorial tree in Ottawa, Canada. His physician, Janet Travell, recommended a rocking-chair, and he installed one in the Oval Office at the White House. Within months, tens of thousands were clamoring for them.

Why is a rocking-chair useful for the person with back pain? Because, as the chair rocks backward and forward, its motion constantly varies the load on the various muscles supporting the upper body. This is important because muscles fatigue quickly if maintained in a fixed position. Rocking constantly varies the tension on a given muscle, which is beneficial.

Be aware, however, that a rocking-chair is *not* a good chair to sit in while motionless. It tilts too far back and soon tires the shoulder and neck muscles.

You will find more on sitting in Chapter 16.

14

Standing

MANY MEN AND WOMEN EARN THEIR LIVING ON their feet. If they suffer chronic back pain, their days can be painful and exhausting.

Most back pain resulting from prolonged standing is a result of bad posture and is avoidable. A reasonably fit person with a healthy back can stand for extended periods without significant discomfort, feeling, at most, moderate fatigue.

But bad posture can transform prolonged standing into an ordeal.

The ideal posture is not as we were told by strict parents: "Stand up straight!" By "straight," the parent meant straining for height, the chin tucked in, the shoulders forced back, the arch of the low back straightened and the knees locked.

You will see the members of a military Honor Guard assume such a stance when they are being reviewed, but it is entirely unnatural and a considerable strain. It is not unusual on a hot day to see a guardsman keel over from a combination of muscular exhaustion and the pooling of blood in the lower extremities, thus depriving the brain.

Maintain a stiffly erect posture for an extended period and it can qualify as a form of torture.

"In my boyhood, my father used to reprove me [Charles Templeton] for what he called my 'round shoulders.' 'For goodness sake, Chuck!' he would say. 'Stand up *straight!*'

"He would then, if I didn't do it quite to his satisfaction, require me to stand for fifteen minutes against the wall: heels touching the baseboard, buttocks, shoulders and the back of my head pressed against the wall.

" 'There, now,' he would say. 'That's the way.'

"It wasn't, of course. It was simply an example of misguided parental bullying. In some obscure way, he may have felt that he was doing his duty; the war had just ended and, because he had five children and a strategically important job he hadn't been required to enlist. 'Stand like a good soldier,' he would call out frequently. (I had often seen off-duty soldiers in the street and they seemed an unkempt lot, indifferent to their posture.)

"Once, his patience worn thin, my father inserted a wooden coat-hanger inside the back of my sweater and made me wear it one full morning as a punishment. It remains one of the vivid memories of my childhood.

"His intentions may have been right; his method was dead wrong and the reasons are obvious. The spine is curved in an elongated S-shape to serve a number of purposes — among them, that it may function as a spring, absorbing impact when necessary.

"Try to straighten out a spring; it requires great effort."

THE IDEAL POSTURE

The ideal posture when standing is not an uncomfortable one. It is one that puts the head directly above the feet and therefore in equilibrium. A vertical line drawn from the ear to the ankle would divide the body's weight exactly in half.

This is not, of course, an inflexible rule. The human body is infinite in its variety and no single guideline applies to everyone. We are a diverse lot and come in all shapes and sizes.

Force the man with that lovingly nurtured beer-belly to "stand up straight" and he would likely strain his back or even tumble forward. There are others who are, for genetic reasons, heavy through the shoulders. If they were forced to maintain the "ideal" posture, it would cause them pain and might do them harm.

But for those average men and women who spend most of the day on their feet, there is no substitute for good posture, and chronic neck and back trouble are often the result of the failure to maintain it.

The best and simplest rule is this: *stand tall — but be at ease.*

THE ABNORMAL ACT OF STANDING ERECT

You may wonder why, when there is nothing organically wrong with your back, standing would give you trouble. It is not difficult to understand.

Think of your body as consisting of four basic segments: the head and neck, the torso, the thighs and the lower extremities.

Each of these segments is attached to the others by what are in effect "muscular hinges." Equilibrium is maintained by signals originating in the inner ear and transmitted to the muscles by the autonomic nervous system. Normally, no conscious thought is required.

But an upright stance is not normal for mammals and is unique in humans — even the apes maintain contact with the ground through their knuckles. It is a posture evolved over millions of years because our progenitors found it advantageous and persisted in trying to achieve it. It was advantageous because it freed their hands for other purposes and because it elevated the head and enabled them to see farther. And being able to see farther made it possible to spot both prey and enemies earlier.

For all its advantages, however, the ability to stand erect has drawbacks. If one's posture is faulty, it can cause undue fatigue. Ideally, the arch of the back, the lordotic curve, should be slightly flattened and the pelvis flexed or tucked under in a modified pelvic tilt. A heavy stomach or weakness in the abdominal muscles tends to arch the back and, in time, can lead to an increasing vulnerability to back problems.

A CONSTANT WAR WITH GRAVITY
The moment you rise to your feet, your body is engaged in an unremitting war with gravity, the force of which is acting to bring you down. You can grasp how constant this tendency is by balancing a stick on the end of a finger. You can maintain the stick in an upright position only by continual adjustments. Just so, your muscles must act to counter the tendency to disequilibrium as you to stand, bend, walk, run, leap, lift and do all the marvelous things of which the human body is capable. This constant monitoring of your equilibrium begins at the feet and works upward, your muscles working to forestall imminent collapse.

At every moment of every day, the forces acting to bring you to the ground must be countered. This, of course, requires energy and, from time to time, fatigued, you must yield by sitting or lying down to rest or sleep.

DEM BONES, DEM BONES, DEM LIVE BONES . . .

When our forbears decided to stand erect, they accepted certain limitations. As marvelous a mechanism as your body is, it doesn't compare with that of most animals in terms of physical capacity. The animals' advantage is, in large part, that they have "four on the floor."

Your six-month-old puppy can outrun you. Give Carl Lewis a 50-meter start in a 100-meter race and any cheetah will overtake him when he is hardly out of the blocks. A Nureyev can leave you thinking you have never seen such physical grace — until you recall watching a gazelle bound across a waterhole.

But, for all its limitations, the human body is, as the Psalmist said, "fearfully and wonderfully made" and serves us magnificently. Essentially, it is a pile of bones (the hip bone connected to the thigh bone, the thigh bone connected to the leg bone . . .), all of which would tumble into an untidy heap were they not bound together and activated by a complex network of nerves, muscles, sinews and tendons.

But, for all the marvels of movement it can accomplish, a given muscle is essentially simple. Consider, as an example, your bicep, the major muscle of the upper arm. When a body-builder (or a growing boy) contracts his bicep and thus bends his arm, he looks with satisfaction (or dismay) at the size and firmness of the bump that appears. That bump is the result of the contraction of the muscle, and its firmness and relative size indicate its strength.

MUSCLE TONE

If a muscle is exercised regularly it acquires what is called muscle tone, a term describing the "fitness" of the muscle in its relaxed state. In a state of fitness, the muscle is ready for use and is capable of meeting such reasonable demands as may be made on it.

However, a muscle that is seldom exercised becomes flaccid and weak and shortened, and when called upon to fulfill its function — especially when fatigued — may tear or rupture in some of its fibers.

Muscles become fatigued for three principal reasons: they have been overstressed, they have been subjected to prolonged emotionally induced tension or they have been maintained in a contracted state for an undue period of time.

An Olympic weight lifter can hoist hundreds of pounds in a sudden explosion of muscular energy. Within seconds, the weight is bulled from the floor, elevated, held for a few seconds and dropped. It is an awesome demonstration of the power of the combined muscles of the body. Afterwards, the muscles are momentarily fatigued, even sore, but the fatigue soon passes and they are ready for the next lift.

Now hand the Olympian a 10-pound weight and ask him to hold it at arm's length for three minutes. The weight may be no more than 2 percent of what he just lifted, but, within a minute, he'll be uncomfortable. Within two minutes he will be grimacing with pain, and before the three minutes has elapsed will probably have lowered his arm.

(Try it yourself with a hardcover book. You'll be squirming within a minute. In two minutes, the pain will be almost unbearable.)

You will grasp how quickly muscle fatigue can occur if you merely clench your fist tightly for thirty seconds. Try it. To descend to trivia, try to hold your eyebrows in an elevated position for one minute. A student remembers sustaining a pose for twenty minutes for an art class —

each student took turns to save the cost of a professional model. Although he was sitting with an elbow on his thigh and his chin resting on his hand, the last five minutes was almost unbearable.

What do these examples indicate? *That muscles in sustained contraction fatigue very quickly.* Muscles don't like to be immobilized, even in the relaxed mode. That's why, even when sitting for an extended period, you have to shift around. That's why, unless you change position in your sleep, your muscles are stiff or sore when you get out of bed in the morning.

Your muscles are particularly vulnerable if immobilized while contracted, and if not soon released will communicate this fact with what can become excruciating pain.

THE PRINCIPLE: STRESS AND RELAX

This principle obtains even when you stand for prolonged periods. Standing, your body is being maintained in an erect position and the operative muscles are essentially immobilized.

That's why it is harder to stand motionless for an hour than it is to walk a mile. When you walk, the muscles of a leg contract when your weight is on it. But, as you move to the other leg, the muscles of the first leg relax. The muscles of each leg are being flexed half the time and relaxed half the time, and fit muscles can do this for hours with little fatigue.

But, when you stand, there is a tendency to remain in one spot and to distribute your weight equally onto both legs, which causes them to tire. Move your weight from one leg to the other in one way or another and the fatigue factor is greatly lessened.

When you must stand for a long time, alter your posture from time to time:

- Set your feet slightly apart and shift your weight from one leg to the other every so often.
- Clasp your hands behind your back for a change or fold them across your chest. Such small changes alter slightly the entire alignment of your body.
- Alternate standing with one foot slightly ahead of the other.
- If you can, stroll about occasionally.
- If feasible, stand with one foot raised and resting on a ledge, a stair, a stool, whatever.
- Put your hands on the back of a chair and transfer some weight to your arms. Try placing a foot on the lowest rung.
- Lean your upper back against a wall. In doing so, you transfer some of your body weight to the wall and remove it from your lower back and legs. While doing so, place your hands behind your lower back and press them against the wall.

You may want to remain limber by trying what is sometimes called "the monkey slump." It is done simply by letting your head, neck, shoulders and arms hang down limply — almost as though the support muscles have given way. Do not lean forward; just slump. Bend your kees slightly at the same time, even let your jaw hang loose. (Wait until you are unobserved, however, because you may look a little goofy.) The brief relaxation so achieved will alter the stress factor in virtually every muscle used in standing and will refresh you. Thirty seconds from time to time is useful.

Don't overdo any one of these aids — they are "helps," not rules. Their purpose is to assist in reducing the stiffness or soreness produced when muscles are contracted but inactive.

Here, indeed, a change *is* as good as a rest.

STANDING IN THE WORKPLACE

Many men and women are required to work while standing at a workbench, a countertop or an assembly-line. If the work surface is at a height that requires constant or frequent bending over (even if slight), there is the likelihood of lower-back fatigue and pain.

It is easy to understand why. The entire torso — approximately half your body weight — is hinged forward at the waist and is being maintained in that position. When you straighten up, the fatigued muscles of the lower back must, literally, lever the torso erect. The farther you are over, the greater the load on your low back muscles. And if the muscles have grown fatigued while maintaining a position, the difficulty increases.

It is a back seizure waiting to happen!

The problem is further intensified if you are overweight or out of shape or getting on in years.

If your work puts you in such a situation, it is imperative that you alter your posture frequently and avoid straightening up suddenly. When, in such a circumstance, back pain strikes, *it is invariably at the moment of the first contraction of the muscles to bring the torso erect*. If you should find yourself in such imminent jeopardy, bend your knees, move your feet forward as far as possible, place your hands on the work surface and *slowly* push yourself erect.

Optionally, if there is a wall or cupboard on the far side of where you are working, assist your return to vertical by extending an arm and pushing against it.

Leaning forward while standing with the knees locked can put as much as 200 pounds of pressure per square inch on the low-back discs, the same amount of pressure as sitting while bent forward.

Hints for the workplace

If you must stand at work, here is a list of postural options you can use to avoid overstressing your back muscles:

- Stand as close as possible to what you are working on.
- Alternately rest one foot or the other on a slightly raised surface — a bottom shelf, a collapsible footrest, a shallow box, even a telephone book will do.
- Stand with one foot alternately ahead of the other.
- Feet in close, lean your pelvic area against the edge of the work surface but don't arch your back excessively in order to do so.
- Shift your weight onto one leg or the other for brief periods.
- If you are using only one hand, place the other on the work surface from time to time and transfer some weight to it.
- Perch on a high stool to take some weight off your feet. And change from one buttock to the other from time to time.

You should use any or all of these options over the course of a day; none of them for extended periods. They will enable you to avoid prolonged immobilization of any particular set of muscles.

THE RIGHT UNDERPINNING

It needs hardly to be mentioned that proper footwear is important if your job requires standing.

Nor need it be emphasized that high heels are a guarantee of back and leg pain, even neck pain — and, of course, sore feet. Most quality shoe stores carry a line of orthopedic shoes, many of them quite modish. You may, however, find the extra expense unnecessary; a good pair of "sensible" shoes with low heels will usually suffice. When you have the option, wear rubber heels. They reduce the impact at the source and can make a considerable difference if you walk or stand frequently on hard surfaces.

If you are having serious trouble with your feet, visit a professional chiropodist or podiatrist. They perform a valuable service. We know of an instance where a chiropodist has, in a single analysis and treatment session, transformed years of torture into permanent relief.

Comfort in your feet is important because, if one or both of your feet is sore, you will try unconsciously to ease the discomfort by altering your normal posture. *Any postural abnormality during prolonged standing can adversely affect your back.*

15

Walking

"WHAT IN THE WORLD IS THE RELATIONSHIP BE-tween cardiovascular exercise and back fitness?"

Legitimate question. The answer is: a great deal.

Fundamental to having a healthy back is having a healthy body. It may be stated as axiomatic that the physically fit have fewer back problems than those who let themselves get out of shape.

Few things could be more obvious: most back problems have an immediate relationship to the condition of the muscles of the back. If your back muscles lack strength or tone, they are more subject to being over-stressed or injured. Regular exercise helps keep muscles fit, and part of any balanced program of exercise is cardiovascular fitness.

Vigorous daily walking is probably the most useful cardiovascular exercise the average person can engage in. No single exercise can match the many benefits it yields, and those benefits are both direct and indirect. It is good for your lungs and heart, and the aerobic aspects are beneficial in a surprising variety of ways. Regular, vigorous walking can improve muscle tone and help reduce the risk of heart disease. It can assist in keeping your weight down and your blood pressure low. It helps also to lessen tension and combat fatigue and can even contribute to meditative thought.

As has been said: "I have but two physicians — my right leg and my left."

Equally important: regular exercise helps in laying down calcium in the bones and keeping them healthy. This is expecially significant for women, who, more than men, tend to suffer osteoporosis as they age.

Specific exercises benefit specific areas of the body. Aerobics benefits the entire body. Oxygen is sent coursing through the veins, invigorating every cell and contributing uniquely to overall fitness.

Beyond that, when you step out purposefully, carry yourself erect, breathe deeply, swing your arms energetically and elevate your heart rate, you not only improve your general fitness, you begin to feel noticeably better about yourself and life in general.

WALKING OR JOGGING?

There is a growing consensus among health experts that, while jogging is indispensable for the athlete in training, it can have negative effects on the average individual seeking simply to improve his or her general fitness level.

Jogging can be particularly deleterious to sufferers from back pain, especially if they carry their fitness-kick to the streets of a large city.

The hard, unyielding pavement transmits shock waves up the legs to the pelvis and lower back and will often distress the joints and muscles. This is particularly true for those individuals who are overweight, for the runner who tends to land heavily on the heels and for the person who is predisposed to back problems.

In most cities there are parklands with paths followed daily by dozens of joggers. One seldom sees them without wondering why they (men and women who are obviously concerned about their health) engage in physical activities so patently detrimental to their bodies.

Study them as they pass. There are as many styles of jogging as there are joggers. Some glide effortlessly with an economy of motion, but the majority lurch, stumble and plod their way along. They seem engaged in self-inflicted torture, in a grim struggle to punish their feet and legs and lungs and heart. Some, their faces distorted and beet-red, seem to be courting a coronary. Others have the pallor of the dead.

Beyond that, when they leave the park to continue their jogging on the streets and sidewalks, you feel that the exhaust-befouled air with which they are filling their lungs will counter any aerobic benefits that might otherwise accrue.

THE RELIGION OF JOGGING

Jogging has become a religion of sorts and, as with most religions, it is only reluctantly criticized.

There can be no doubt that jogging can contribute to cardiovascular health (one would be a fool to inveigh against it) but, as commonly indulged in, it is anything but a carefree jaunt down the road to fitness. And, not least — this being our concern here — it can be bad for your back.

If while jogging you feel the impact of your heels on the ground transferring up your legs to the pelvis and low back, even to your head and neck, you should give thought as to whether the presumed benefits of the exercise don't need to be reappraised.

Jogging for miles each day on an unyielding surface, you even risk creating tiny stress-fractures in the vertebrae and could find yourself permanently sidelined. The multiple impacts won't do the knee and hip joints much good either.

A friend, an avid jogger who has run anywhere from 3 to 10 miles a day for years, began to have pains in a knee joint and, following the run, pains in the back. When the symptoms persisted and worsened, he sought professional help and ended up having arthroscopic surgery. It was not successful. He has substituted daily walks and cycling and, happily, the symptoms have disappeared.

If after jogging, you regularly feel back pain — and not necessarily *immediately* afterwards — you would be well advised to consult a professional and might be well advised to stop.

You should also examine your style. Perhaps you are swinging your arms across your body. This can produce torque in your lower trunk, which, repeated ten thousand times, can stress the facet joints whose function in the lumbar region includes containing excessive twisting.

Even the aerobobic benefits of jogging become questionable if, for an hour or two each day, you inhale the noxious fumes of the passing traffic. If, however, you are determined to continue your daily program of jogging, wear the best shock-absorbing shoes you can buy and, if necessary, drive to an area that will get you off the streets.

A better option is to switch to vigorous walking. You will benefit as much aerobically, and it will be easier on the joints, the muscles and the back.

WALKING — THE BETTER WAY

If you decide to begin a regimen of daily walking, take the time first to get fitted with a proper pair of shoes.

There is little to choose between the shoes made by the better-known manufacturers. Go to a store that specializes in sporting equipment (these days, some are veritable emporiums) but be judicious. Don't buy the pair that first comes to hand simply because the shoes bear a familiar trademark or are purportedly worn by a famous athlete.

There are literally dozens of specialized shoes on the market, some especially designed for walking. They differ in construction from jogging shoes, and you should see to it that you get what you need. Not uncommonly, a salesperson — even in a major sporting-goods store — will insist that there is no significant difference between jogging and walking shoes. There is. Tell the salesperson precisely what you are looking for and how you will use them. And, before making your purchase, put on *both* shoes and stride about the store for a few minutes.

The wrong salesperson can literally get you off on the wrong foot.

THE FREQUENCY OF WALKING

How often should you walk? A minimum of four days a week. You may wish to walk every day, and if you do, do so. Most experts suggest, however, that four days will yield as many benefits as seven, so suit your convenience.

How far and how fast should you walk? That depends on your age, your level of fitness, your weight, the condition of your back and the way your body reacts to exercise. If you have any doubts about your heart or feel any adverse effects after exercise, check it out.

The ideal pace for walking is to walk so that you have the feeling you are spinning the earth a little with each stride.

MONITORING YOUR HEART RATE

Because the reader of these pages could be unfit or unwell or aging, a word of counsel about the stress that vigorous walking may impose on an unhealthy or aging heart. There is a generally accepted standard for improving physical fitness — *Exercise sufficiently to raise your heartbeat into the beneficial range for twenty minutes, three or four times a week*.

And how can you judge the beneficial range, especially when it changes as you grow older? Here is a simple measure:

Take your age.

Subtract it from 210.

Calculate 75 percent of the remainder.

EXAMPLE: You are 50. Subtract it from 210 and the remainder is 160. 75 percent of 160 is 120. Normally, that is your beneficial range.

This means that, after warming up through the first three to five minutes, you should be walking with sufficient vigor to maintain your heart rate at close to your individual maximum and should sustain it at that level for the next fifteen minutes.

When you begin, use common sense and don't overdo it. If you are going to err one way or another, do it on the side of caution. If you feel pain or discomfort in the chest, arm, neck or jaw, stop and check with your doctor. Don't overstress yourself first time out. Increase your workout daily to where you reach a level that taxes but doesn't exhaust you.

Bear in mind that you need to work at it to get any

benefit from it. Going for a stroll may be pleasant but it will do your heart and lungs and muscles little good.

You will know without anyone's counsel whether you are pampering or punishing yourself. Neither is desirable. Go at it too hard and, rather than do you good, it may harm you. Coddle yourself, and the entire program is a waste of time.

When you return from your walk you should be fatigued but not pooped.

BENEFITING THE UPPER BODY

If you want to extend the benefits of walking to your upper body, do as boxers do when training for a fight. They shadow-box as they log their many miles, throwing punches at the air. You, too, may find it useful: good for the arms, shoulders, bust, stomach and back.

But a word of caution: don't fantasize about becoming a Sugar Ray Leonard and overdo it. And throw jabs not hooks — at least in the beginning. You don't want to throw yourself off balance or unduly stress your facet joints.

A further note: Walking on paths through parks or across the uneven surfaces of open terrain, you are always at risk of stumbling, and this is particularly true for the person who wears bifocals. Better to work out without them. Wearing them, it is easy to misjudge a tiny ridge or a shallow step or trip over the exposed root of a tree. Everyone has had the experience of "that extra step that isn't there." Your nervous system is not anticipating the drop, and the unexpected impact can sent a severe jolt through the ankles and knees and up the spine.

Such a misstep is jarring for anyone; it can be especially painful, even damaging, for the person with a bad back.

BEWARE: CHILDREN AND DOGS

When returning from a walk, beware of children and dogs.

When children and dogs see Mummy or Daddy or the Adored Owner come in sight, they are liable to run toward you in great excitement and, respectively, leap into your arms or jump up against you.

We are acquainted with a man who was recovering from a prolonged session of back spasms and finally felt up to going for a walk. Returning to the house, he was congratulating himself on how well the venture had gone, until his Labrador retriever went into ecstatic excitement at seeing his master out of doors again and put him on his back on the lawn, howling in pain.

THE HABIT OF WALKING

A regular program of walking can do you worlds of good and possibly extend your life. In the context of this book it can help combat what is commonly called "nagging backache," particularly when it is induced by tension.

Begin regular walking; it may very well accomplish more than a trip to the therapist.

16

Driving Your Car

SUCH ARE THE DISTANCES FROM WORK IN TODAY'S sprawling cities that it is not uncommon for a suburbanite to spend two or more hours each weekday behind the wheel of a car. Much of that time is spent idling or barely moving in traffic, in circumstances rife with stress and almost guaranteed to induce tension:

- You are running late.
- The visibility is bad.
- The road surface is wet or icy.
- There is the inevitable "Construction Zone" up ahead.
- Other drivers are acting obnoxiously.
- Problems at work or at home are nagging you.
- You are low on fuel with the next exit miles ahead.
- Moreover, the uneven surfaces of the road seem to be transferring to your back with more than their usual impact.

For all its convenience, traveling by car can be something of an ordeal. For the driver of a truck, his back a locus of pain, it can be a daily torment — with no solution in sight.

A HOSTILE ENVIRONMENT

The automobile is a part of nearly everyone's daily life, and women drive as often as men. Unfortunately, the driver's seat in many cars — and certainly in most trucks — can be a hostile environment.

- It is awkward to get into and out of the driver's seat.
- The seat back slants at an uncomfortable angle.
- The bench seat tends to fall off toward the middle.
- The steering wheel, the controls and the foot pedals are awkwardly placed and hard to reach.
- For shorter men and women, the line of sight is a problem and a cause of straining.

Fortunately, much can be done to resolve most of these problems and make the time spent in your car a pleasure rather than an ordeal.

Let us begin with certain basics.

POSITIONING THE CAR SEAT

As was noted to earlier, a much-quoted Swedish study on posture demonstrated that the pressures on the discs of the lower back are greater when sitting than when standing, and even greater when leaning forward while sitting. Inasmuch as this is often the posture assumed in driving a car, it is little wonder that many men and women with back problems find their condition aggravated while driving — or afterwards.

This finding may come as something of a surprise. You may feel that you are most relaxed when at ease in the well-upholstered seat of your car — and you may be. You may well insist that you feel more comfortable with the seat tilted well back — and this may be so for brief periods

— but on an extended trip, with the road bumps being transferred directly to your lower back, you may have cause to revise that opinion.

To correct the problem, set the car seat as far forward as is convenient without your being cramped or your ability to operate the brakes and gas pedal impaired. If the back of the seat is adjustable, tilt it forward until it is close to vertical — ideally, it should slant back at no more than ten degrees. Not least, you will not have constantly to bend forward to grasp the steering wheel. Moreover, it will put your knees higher than your hips, which is advantageous.

There are a number of other things you can do to to counter a badly engineered seat. Purchase one of those rectangular, wedge-shaped cushions available in automobile stores, and position it, either behind your back or under the buttocks. Some are available with an elastic strap that holds them in position on the back of the seat. The Obus Forme support may prove beneficial. Some of the upper price-range cars come equipped with an orthopedic seat. Some automobile accessory manufacturers make a special lumbar seat, but they are expensive. If your work requires you to spend much of your day in your car, it may be worth the investment.

Short of this, take particular trouble to see that you settle into your seat as comfortably as possible under the circumstances. Don't slump. Sit up straight and shove your tailbone against the seat back. If the design of the seat still leaves you tilted back, modify it with a small cushion, a piece of foam rubber, even a folded bath towel. Incorrect posture while driving can quickly lead to back discomfort.

SMALL PROBLEM; SERIOUS CONSEQUENCES

"I [Templeton] was a passenger in a taxi some years ago. The driver, noticing that I had entered the cab in a circumspect fashion, said, 'Bad back, huh?'

" 'Just being careful,' I said.

" 'Let me tell you about *my* back,' he said.

"I groaned inwardly but said nothing, realizing that, a captive audience, I was going to hear his story whether I wanted to or not.

" 'I only drive a hack in the winter,' he continued. 'Summers I drive one of them big tractor-trailer rigs coast to coast, but it's too dangerous in winter.'

" 'Uh huh,' I murmured.

" 'The funny thing is,' he said, warming to his story, 'I used to get a bad back every summer. It didn't make sense. I was working shorter hours, the weather was better and I didn't have to cope with city traffic.

" 'I went to every kind of doctor,' he continued, 'and none of them could figure out why I had this problem in summer but not in the winter. I finally wangled it through my family doctor to talk to a specialist. Maybe you've heard of him.' He mentioned a name. I mumbled something that could be taken for a yes or no and he continued.

" 'He's supposed to know more about back pain than anybody; I mean the guy's a real expert. He couldn't work me in for an appointment but he agreed to talk to me on the phone. I told him the problem and, when I finished, he asked me what I thought was a dumb question: 'Where do you carry your wallet?' 'When I'm driving taxi,' I said, 'I keep it locked in the glove compartment so, if I should get held up, all the guy will get is what's in my pocket. On the road I keep it in my hip pocket so I got money when I stop to eat.'

"He swiveled his neck around to look at me. 'You'll never guess what he said.'

" 'I have no idea,'

" 'Without another question, the Doc said, 'With that wallet in your hip pocket, you're bouncing along all day with your spine tilted out of line. Take it out of your hip pocket and carry it somewheres else.'

" 'I did what he said,' the cabbie concluded, 'and I've never had a problem since.' "

Out of such slight postural misalignments can major problems grow. It is never more true than when you are driving.

GETTING INTO AND OUT OF THE CAR

A common problem for the sufferer from back pain is getting into and out of the car.

It can be a complex and sometimes painful undertaking, especially if you are relatively tall or overweight. Getting into the car necessitates bending over, ducking your head, twisting your torso and shifting your entire body weight while seated — all difficult moves when your back is in a dicey state. Getting out can be almost as awkward.

How can such problems be minimized?

First, by planning ahead. You can simplify the problem if, in leaving the car, you prepare it for the next time you will use it. Park in a place that will permit you, when you return, to open the door wide. In your garage this may mean removing anything that will be in the way of the opening door. If you park in a double garage it may mean changing your usual parking position. If you park in a single garage, the configuration of the interior may make it wise to back in rather than drive in.

If you do back in and have passed your middle years, take care not to twist your torso excessively while trying to determine when you have reached the back wall. Aging spines are subject to diminished torsion flexibility and the facet joints can react adversely to frequent twisting. Instead, make a mark on the garage wall beside your front door indicating where the car should be when parked, and simply line up with that.

Each time you get out of the car, leave the seat fully retracted. If you have tilt-steering, leave the wheel in the elevated position. This will not only facilitate your getting out of the car, it will make it easier to get in.

Preparing to get in, set the door in the fully open position and stand with your back to the seat, the back of your legs close to the doorsill. Then — your left hand on the back of the seat and your right hand holding onto the inside edge of the open door — simply lower yourself onto the edge of the seat.

Now, reach up with your left hand and take hold of the roof edge. Put your right hand behind you on the car seat and, lifting most of your weight, pivot your body to the right, settling behind the steering wheel.

There are two cautions to be observed: 1. If you are tall, you may have to bend your neck forward to pass beneath the roof edge and that can be painful. Bend your knees and do it slowly. 2. In making the turn to settle behind the wheel, do not twist. Move your body as a unit.

Getting out of the car, move the seat as far back as possible, tilt the steering wheel into the up position and open the door wide. Now, reverse the actions you took getting into the car — remembering again to move the body as a unit and to avoid twisting.

PUBLIC PARKING LOTS

In a public parking lot, look for a space that will enable you to open the door fully. You can make this easier by parking slightly off center, to the right of your allocated space. In fairness, do not make your neighbor's access difficult. (Not least because he may reciprocate by banging his door handle against your paint job or by bending your radio antenna.)

If possible, find a spot with a wall or pillar to your left. You can thus guarantee easy access to your car when you return.

You will have to be the judge as to the wisdom of the following suggestion, but if your back is in a condition where any abnormal bending or twisting may precipitate a serious problem, park in one of the spaces reserved for the handicapped. Leave a note under the windshield explaining your action. Authenticated by some credible medical evidence, your action will probably be accepted as legitimate in the event you do get a summons.

If getting into and out of your car poses a major problem, apply for a license permitting you to park in the zones reserved for the handicapped. Again, you may be required to present a letter from your doctor.

THE STRESS OF DRIVING

As mentioned earlier, driving a car can be surprisingly stressful. One thing you can do to reduce that stress is to control your emotions when behind the wheel.

An odd psychological transformation overtakes many of us (more men than women) when we get behind the wheel of a car. People who are normally civil and restrained become competitive, reckless and boorish. Their rudeness stimulates a response-in-kind, and the whole sequence accelerates.

We have no data to subtantiate it but think it likely that there are few activities that raise blood pressure so high, so often, as driving on congested highways.

It can, literally, give you a pain in the neck — *and* shoulders *and* back. If you find yourself tense while driving, work out a relaxation pattern you can use. Here is a simple one:

- If you frequently find your shoulders drawn up taut, rotate them for thirty seconds and then, *consciously*, lower them.
- If your neck is stiff or painful, draw your chin in slowly while reaching upward with the crown of your head. Hold for a count of five and repeat.
- Turn your head from side to side *in slow motion*, as though saying no. Follow that by nodding a number of times, as though saying yes. (Wait until you're stopped or barely moving, of course.)
- Tilt your head sideways, as though trying to rest an ear on your shoulder — both sides. Do not strain. Hold for a count of five and repeat.
- You may feel foolish following this final suggestion but, one by one, specifically naming them, order each of your major muscles to grow slack. ("Okay, neck muscles, relax! Sink between the shoulders. *Down!* . . . Now, right shoulder, your turn. Sag . . . Droop . . . *Down boy!*") As your mind ranges over your body, visualize more and more of your body weight depressing the seat beneath you.

If your drive is a long one, move the seat back for a few minutes from time to time in order to alter your posture — only, of course, when you are stopped in traffic or moving at a crawl.

Finally, if you tend to be an intense or competitive type (and many sufferers with back problems are), make a conscious decision not to get steamed up by other drivers, whatever the provocation. Leave off cursing or shaking your fist or retaliating in kind.

Could lower the blood pressure, too!

UNLOADING THE CAR

Driving a car can be stressful; loading and unloading it can be downright hazardous.

We use our cars to transport ourselves; we use them almost as often to transport things: bassinets and strollers, bags filled with supermarket food, sacks of lawn-fertilizer, gardening equipment, briefcases and luggage — anything and everything that will fit into the trunk.

The only catch is that what goes in must come out, and for the man or woman guarding a bad back, there are few places as booby-trapped with risk as a car trunk.

The basic rule in lifting is to get your feet as close to the object as possible and then raise it vertically. The farther an object is from your body, the greater the load on your low-back muscles when you try to raise it.

"Fine," you say. "But how do you get an object stowed in an automobile trunk close to your body? And how do you get your feet positioned close to it?"

The fact *is*, there *is* no easy way, and there are no simple solutions. These suggestions will help:

• Begin by removing the objects closest to you. Before removing them, drag them as near to you as possible. Continue to do this with each object to be removed. In pulling the farthest objects toward you, use one arm only. As you lean over, support the weight of your torso with the other arm, placing your hand on the edge of the trunk or on any other stable place available.

• You may find it useful, when leaning forward, to place one knee on top of the rear bumper. Experiment.

THE TWO-LIFT LIFT

When lifting heavy objects from the trunk, do not do it alone if help is available. If it must be done alone, *don't do it in a single lift.*

On the first lift, rest the object on the rim of the trunk and steady it there while you position yourself for the second lift. This is crucial. The object is now higher and closer to you and can easily be carried away.

A particularly difficult challenge is lifting a large object or a small child from the back seat of a two-door car. Avoid it if possible by reserving the right front seat for the child or for large packages. Older children or adult passengers can sit in back.

If you have no option but to place heavy objects in the back seat, again use two lifts rather than one, temporarily resting the load on the folded front seat and then positioning yourself advantageously for the second lift.

DRIVING ON THE VERGE

You may sometime find yourself forced by circumstances to drive while your back is in danger of spasm. If you can avoid it, do so. If you must persevere, exercise caution.

A patient recalls having to travel a considerable distance on the streets of a large city during rush-hour. He was enduring severe pain in his low back, and experience told him that he was in immediate danger of suffering a muscle spasm. He weighed all his options and decided for a number of reasons that, despite the jeopardy, he would continue on to the safe harbor of his home.

He knew that a bad seizure could possibly render him unable to come to a safe stop. He knew also that a car seat is not the ideal place in which to be confined during such a problem. So he moved into the right lane, slowed, put on his flasher-lights and kept a constant lookout ahead for a service station, a drive-in or a side street, any place into which he might pull if the worst happened.

He made it safely home but realized in retrospect that he had acted foolishly. It would have been wiser to have pulled into a service station and parked out of the flow of traffic. There, he could try to relax, wait out the crisis, perhaps even lie down on the seat. And, if bad came to worst, he could blow his horn and get someone's attention.

If you feel you are in immediate danger of a back seizure and believe it might be incapacitating, pull over as soon as feasible. If you are on a highway, park on the shoulder or, better, take the first off-ramp and seek help. Otherwise, you may find yourself forced to wait indefinitely until a police car chances to come along.

In the unlikely event you face such a serious emergency, the best option is to pull over, park and put on your flashers. If you have something at hand like a handkerchief, a scarf, a necktie or whatever, put an arm out of the window and wave it.

17

Stress, Tension and Fear

IN AN EPISODE IN THE LATE WALT KELLY'S POPU-
lar comic strip, *Pogo*, Pogo says, "We have met the enemy and it is us."

No sentiment could be more appropriate when you
examine the causes of recurring back pain. Usually, the
victim is his or her own worst enemy, and the primary
reason for that individual's self-induced problem is
tension.

Emotional tension is the cause of the majority of back
problems. A chronically tense muscle becomes fatigued.
It loses much of its flexibility. It cannot react as it should
and, subjected to sudden stress, is likely to rupture or go
into spasm.

A TENSION-RIDDEN SOCIETY

Muscular tension is a byproduct of our contemporary
way of life.

The pressures impinging on most of us stem from our
lifestyle and from the stressful world we inhabit. It is

revelatory that back pain is particularly prevalent in the Western democracies. Indeed, the problem has become epidemic. It ranks second (after colds and influenza) as the largest cause of workforce absenteeism in the United States, Canada, Great Britain and Sweden. It has been estimated that 60 to 80 percent of the population suffers from back pain at some time in life. On any working day in North America, approximately seven million people are incapacitated because of back problems, most of them in the low back.

Moreover, the problems affect men and women almost equally.

Many are made tense by the circumstances of their work, by the pressures to succeed, by the desire to increase their income, by family problems, by the demands of competition and by feelings of guilt over their sometime failure to be a caring parent, a thoughtful spouse, a good citizen.

Others are made tense by the twin pressures of competing at work and running a home, by the unremitting demands of children, by social obligations, by the need to remain youthful and attractive, by financial strictures.

THE STRESSED INDIVIDUAL

The stresses of our contemporary way of life have a way of lodging in the neck and shoulders and lower back, of drawing muscles taut and setting one up as a candidate for either a first back seizure or a repetition of the bouts of pain endured in previous years.

Many sufferers from back pain live under the shadow of their affliction, fearing another attack. Fear creates stress, and stress creates muscle-tension; the combination may radically alter one's life.

- It can alter posture. Doctors are familiar with the back patient who shuffles into the office, torso bent forward, a hand pressed to the back, a knitted frown between the eyebrows.

- It can lessen physical activity. Participation in sports falls off. "I'd love to join you but I wouldn't dare. Just nine holes — are you kidding? One dubbed tee-shot and I'd be in bed for a week."
- It provides an excuse for staying home, for not attending that symphony concert, not going to that tedious party, not making that social call. "I'd like to, but the old back won't take it."
- It provides a justification for laziness. "Darling, I want to clean out the garage — you know that. And I sure could use the exercise. But it would put me back in bed, and do you want that? As a matter of fact, I think I'll go lie down for a few minutes."
- It can even militate against taking a vacation. "Man! Could I use one! But I don't sleep well in hotel beds. And all that walking! ... First thing you know, I'll put my back out and end up in some god-forsaken hospital where they don't speak English."
- It can sabotage a couple's sex life. "Not tonight, darling. I've got a backache."

No matter how it may be disguised, the villain of the piece is fear. And the product of that fear is increased tension.

THE TENSION-PRONE INDIVIDUAL

One of the more familiar statements in books dealing with back problems is the assertion: "Once a person has had a back injury, he or she is four times more likely to have a second one."

As with many statistically based conclusions, this one is both true and false. It may be a statistical fact but it is nonsense unless this qualification is added: The initial

back injury does not itself make you likely to suffer another; *you are likely to suffer another because you are
the kind of person you are.*

If you are subject to frequent back problems, it is probable that you are a person whose emotions play a dis-
proportionately large part in your life. Authoritative
studies have shown that more than 80 percent of patients with back pain have a history of such emotion-
related illnesses as migraine, chronic headache, heartburn, nervous problems, stomach ulcers, spastic colon
and certain allergies.

If you are particularly given to tension and anxiety, it is
likely that you will be subject to back problems.

THE HELPING HAND THAT DOESN'T

We recognize the familiar image of the sufferer from back
pain who stands with both hands pressed against the
low back. Surely it is obvious that the posture is accomplishing the opposite of what is intended.

The hands pressed against the back are a prop. The
muscles of the arms are being employed to ease the load
on the muscles of the back. It may be good for the arms; it
is bad for the back. The very muscles that need to be
strengthened by use are being weakened by disuse.
Soon, muscle tone diminishes and the potential for a
serious problem increases.

Why does the individual who assumes such a posture
do so? The answer is obvious: to lessen or to avoid pain. It
may achieve this temporarily, but it is a benefit likely to
worsen the problem.

The individual is supporting the back muscles because
they are weak, and in doing so is making them weaker.
What needs to be done is to make them stronger, and this
can be achieved only by correcting the posture and en-
gaging in regular exercise.

FEAR AND BAD POSTURE

The fear of a back attack can induce a back attack. Worrying about it can lead to bad posture, and bad posture can lead to any number of physical ills — sore muscles, fatigue, a variety of related pains and, finally, back problems.

It is normal for the individual suffering back pain to try to ease the discomfort by altering his or her posture. The pain is dominant on the right side, so you compensate by easing the load on the muscles on that side. This puts the entire upper body out of alignment and results in the corresponding muscles on the other side reacting to the extra demands by tensing. Time passes, these muscles grow stronger, their counterparts weaken, the imbalance becomes fixed and the problem is now serious. In the meantime, the strain on the overloaded muscles can lead to chronic problems.

THE "WHAT IF?" SYNDROME

We call the fear felt by chronic back pain sufferers "apprehension tension." It might well be called the "What if?" syndrome.

- *What if* I bend over to tie my shoelace and can't straighten up?
- *What if* I slip in the shower or get trapped in the bathtub?
- *What if* I lift the baby out of the playpen and have a spasm?
- *What if* I try this exercise and pull a muscle?
- *What if* I mow the lawn and put my back out?
- *What if* I get an attack when I'm out of town and can't get home?
- *What if?* . . . *What if?* . . .

There is a mystique about the back that contributes to its negative impact on the psyche. Sprain an ankle and, after the initial pain has passed, you will treat it as an inconvenience. You may hobble about, wrap the ankle in an elastic bandage, prop it on a footstool when you sit, rent a crutch for a few days and even make jokes about the resident cripple. But it won't intimidate and depress you; it is more a major inconvenience than a major affliction.

A sprained muscle in your back is not, essentially, a very different thing from a sprained ankle. Unfortunately, however, the victim may all-too-willingly take to his or her bed, load up on analgesics, don a put-upon expression, walk as though on eggs and immediately limit daily activities. He or she not only complains constantly about the problem, but thinks black thoughts. And more often than not those thoughts are not normal everyday fretting; they are something deeper. There is a touch of primal fear.

FEAR: THE ENEMY

Much of the fear the back-pain sufferer feels derives from the location of the pain. The spine (with the heart, the eye and the brain) is thought of as one of the particularly vulnerable parts of the body. Cut a finger or gash a knee and you treat it with a dab of peroxide and a BandAid. But experience a pain in your chest, and you react differently: you feel a touch of panic until you are sure it is merely heartburn. Similarly, suffer a sharp twinge in your lower back, and you freeze with apprehension.

Nor are these unreasonable fears: heart trouble can leave you dead, eye problems can leave you blind, brain damage can leave you a vegetable and a serious back injury can leave you incapacitated.

THE DURABLE SPINE

But, for all its fragile appearance, the spine is an astonishingly durable part of the body. Look at a plaster-cast model of it and it suggests a Rube Goldberg contraption — a pile of oddly shaped bones maintained in precarious balance. It is anything but that. The evidence of its resilient toughness fills medical files.

Let us take a moment to reinforce that fact: men and women have survived plane crashes, where the plane has been totaled and passengers have been killed, with few if any back injuries among the survivors. Workmen have fallen from tall structures, breaking both legs and the pelvis, without injuring the spine. The old and the very young have tumbled from highrise apartment balconies without suffering any major back trauma. Other bones may be fractured, internal injuries may be sustained, severe gashes may be inflicted but, surprisingly often, the back is undamaged.

So if you are subject to intimidating fears about the fragility of your back, put the thought away. Your back may pain you, it may inconvenience or immobilize you, it may limit you and, in rare cases, even cripple you, but the great majority of back troubles pose no problems of consequence.

So forsake your unreasonable anxiety. If it stimulates you to treat your back sensibly, the fear is useful. If it dogs your days and creates constant anxiety, it is harmful.

Worse, the fear may itself make some of your fears come true.

A PROBLEM YOU CAN DEAL WITH

There are many specific causes of back trouble but essentially only five basic categories: those resulting from injury, those in which there is a physiological abnormality, those stemming from disease or aging, those resulting from faulty body-mechanics and those resulting from the stresses of our contemporary way of life.

There is little you can do to avoid the physiological problems — those resulting from disease or congenital deformity, the aging process or accidents — but, fortunately, they are the minority. The vast majority of back problems stem from emotional stress, tension, fatigue, work-related injuries, the inability to make decisions in times of pressure, poor posture, pregnancy, overdone sports activity, and obesity, and they are all within the control of the sufferer.

- You *can* deal with tension.
- You *can* diminish your emotional stress.
- You *can* guard against fatigue.
- You *can* correct bad posture.
- You *can* be sensible in playing sports.
- You *can* protect yourself from injuries on the job.

To be a person subject to back problems and not take the steps available to avoid recurrent attacks is to be foolish in the extreme.

TENSION-AWARENESS

The best place to begin is to heighten your awareness about the essential facts relating to tension. Realize that tension resides in the mind. It originates in your thoughts or emotions and manifests itself in your body. Consequently, it must be dealt with there.

Not least, you can begin to increase your sensitivity to the onset of stress. A number of early-warning symptoms signal that tension is building within you. They include:

- irritability,
- a hair-trigger temper,
- the sense of being drawn taut,
- an inner trembling,
- an upset stomach,
- chronic fatigue,

- tightness in the neck and shoulders,
- pain at the center of the back,
- nagging pain in the low back.

To disregard these indications of stress, to let them build over a period of time and do nothing to counter them, is to invite trouble — particularly when there are techniques available to combat them.

We deal in the next chapter with some of the ways in which you can rid yourself of chronic tension and thus nullify its effects.

18

Releasing Tension

TENSION ORIGINATES IN THE MIND AND MANIFESTS itself in the muscles. It is released through thought, muscular activity and controlled breathing.

In order to release tension by proper breathing, it is essential to know the mechanics of the breathing process.

Breathing is one of the few body functions that is controlled by both the brain and the autonomic nervous system. We normally breathe about sixteen times a minute when inactive, but the rate is affected by a number of external and internal factors, among them, temperature changes, body movement and stress.

Breathing is the process by which air is brought into the lungs and thereby in contact with the blood. When we inhale, the muscles attached to the ribs and the diaphragm expand the chest cavity in all three dimensions by raising the ribcage and lowering the diaphragm. This creates an area of relatively low pressure. The air then rushes in and inflates the lungs. As it does, the blood is "recharged" as the oxygen is exchanged for carbon dioxide and vaporized water.

When we exhale, the muscles are relaxed and the carbon dioxide and vaporized water are drawn from the lungs by the lower atmospheric pressure outside the body.

But breathing fulfills a second important function: it is an important means of relaxation.

BREATHING AND RELAXATION

It is our view that the pattern of breathing commonly advocated for relaxation is counterproductive. The instruction given is to take a series of slow, prolonged inhalations, entirely filling the lungs, hold the air for a moment and then slowly and completely empty the lungs.

This is an excellent way to oxygenate the blood, but it is not relaxing. Indeed, it has the opposite effect. The freshly oxgenated blood, rather than relax the muscles and the mind, tends to invigorate both.

Learning from nature

In seeking the proper technique for relaxation through breathing, it is useful to study nature.

Observe how an animal breathes when it wants to relax. Watch your dog when he lies down to sleep. He puts his head down, takes a long, deep breath and then simply releases it. Note that the exhalation is not slow and controlled, it is almost a collapse of the lungs. Often, at the end of a single exhalation, the dog is asleep.

Now analyze the bio-mechanics of yawning. A yawn is an involuntary action; you yawn when you are tired. It is nature's way of relaxing you, of preparing you for sleep.

But note what happens when you yawn. You take a slow, deep breath, your mouth and the back of your throat fully open. Often, as the inhalation concludes, there are one or two slight "catches" of breath — nature's way of filling the lungs completely.

The exhalation is, however, entirely unlike the inhalation. It is *not* a controlled process; it is — as we observed in the dog — almost a collapse of the muscles of the diaphragm. As the lungs empty, the shoulders and ribcage come down, and there is a clearly evident release of tension in the muscles of the chest, shoulders and arms.

A further example: observe your involuntary reaction when you have narrowly averted some danger or escaped from a frightening predicament. How does your body react? To release the tension created by the experience, you draw a deep breath and expel it with a whoosh, usually saying something like "Whew!"

It is through this relaxation of the diaphragm that our bodies reduce muscular tension.

Relaxation breathing
The key to relaxation breathing is breathing out. The reason is obvious — it takes energy to inhale but none to exhale. When you take a breath, the muscles of the diaphragm must be drawn down and the ribcage elevated. But exhaling requires no energy — merely the relaxation of the muscles involved.

Conversely, when you practice controlled deep-breathing, the muscles of the diaphragm are tensed through the entire cycle and no relaxation benefit is achieved.

Pause in your reading for a moment to impress on yourself how fundamental this "collapse exhalation" is to relaxation.

Take a deep breath. Slowly fill your lungs to their full capacity and then exhale. But don't exhale in a slow controlled way; simply let the muscles of your diaphragm relax. Note that, as this happens, the muscles of the back, shoulders, neck and arms also tend to relax.

If you want to learn to relax, learn relaxation breathing. Using relaxation breathing, you do what nature intends: you draw in a slow, deep breath, and when the lungs are filled, simply let go, allowing the exhalation to happen. Don't try to assist the process; *simply let it happen*.

Yawn breathing

You may find it useful to go beyond this and to develop the ability to do what we call "yawn-breathing." Nothing to it; it is simply controlled yawning.

Here's how: inhale slowly and deeply. While doing so, open your mouth wide and, simultaneously, *open the back of your throat as wide as you can*. After a try or two you will find that your autonomic nervous system will take over and convert the inhalation into an involuntary yawn.

You have heard the saying "Yawning's catching." Imitate the physiological actions of a yawn and you will yawn.

Practice it. *Think* yawn, and as you do, open the back of your throat. You will soon discover that you can induce a yawn any time you want to. Moreover, you will find that, usually, a second yawn will follow the first almost automatically.

No exercise will more effectively relax the upper body than a short series of great yawns.

Optionally, you may wish to experiment with another breathing technique, one used by hypnotherapists to induce total relaxation: draw a prolonged, deep breath, simultaneously slowly rolling your eyeballs upward. When your lungs are filled to capacity and your eyes are turned upward in the sockets as far as they will go, release the air and slowly roll your eyeballs downward — *coinciding the two actions*.

Sounds complicated, but it isn't. Some find it very effective.

MIND AND BODY RELAXATION

Here now is a series of simple exercises that will enable you to reduce the tension in your body and your mind and thus lessen the likelihood of recurring back attacks.

There are two excellent places in which to learn and use the techniques: your bed or an easy chair. It must be some place where you can relax and will not be interrupted. The ideal place is your bedroom. The ideal time may be just before sleep.

Begin by getting comfortable. Lie on your back, legs outstretched, arms alongside your body but free of it — whatever feels comfortable. Loosen or remove any restricting clothing. Position a shallow pillow under your head. If it is daytime, draw the drapes or close your eyes.

If you are doing the exercises in an easy chair, slump and make yourself as comfortable as possible. Loosen any tight clothing. Spread your legs comfortably and rest your hands, palms up, fingers loosely bent between your upper thighs. Close your eyes and let your head tilt forward — not excessively, just enough that you are not supporting it.

When you are ready, begin the relaxation process with two or, at most, three yawn-breaths — no more, we don't want a lot of deep breathing. At the end of each breath, take note of the tension draining from your muscles; you will be able to feel it.

You are now ready to begin work on relaxing each section of the body in sequence. This is done by tensing the muscles of the various areas for five seconds, releasing and moving on to the next.

Hugging yourself

Begin with an exercise designed to relax *all* the muscles of your upper body. Wrap your arms about your upper torso as far as they will go. Each hand should be close to or actually on your shoulder blades. Raise your shoulders as you do this and pull your neck down. Now hug yourself. Tightly! Hold it for a slow count of five ("One thousand, two thousand, three thousand, etc.") and release.

As you release, totally relax. Let your arms lie slack on the bed or, if you are in a chair, between your thighs. Concentrate on the sense that all the muscles of your upper body are resting after their effort.

The neck and shoulder muscles

Tension often localizes in the neck. Occasionally, during a time of stress or anxiety, you may have found yourself with a stiff or sore neck, the pain often radiating out to the shoulders and upper back. You may have noticed also that, under pressure, we tend to raise our shoulders slightly and to draw in the neck — perhaps a reflex from the days when our primitive ancestors hunkered down and sought to make themselves small in times of danger.

We begin our series of relaxation exercises with the neck, gently rolling the head back and forth on the pillow. Don't strain or tighten the muscles; let them go slack. This is just for limbering up. Continue for perhaps ten seconds.

Now, facing forward, draw your chin in as close to your neck as possible while, at the same time, reaching upward with the crown of your head. Hold for a slow count of five and release.

Now, tilt (tilt, don't turn) your head far to the right as though trying to touch your ear to your shoulder. Slowly. Hold for five seconds and release. *Do not* try to make ear and shoulder meet — you could pull a muscle in your neck — merely exert firm but not extreme pressure. Repeat, turning the left side.

Now, *turn* your head to the right — slowly. Do not strain to go to the limit; turn until it begins to hurt. Now, do the same to the left. A count of five in each case, and release. If your pillow hinders movement, get rid of it.

The shoulders and chest

Bring your shoulders as far forward as they will go and hold them there for a full five seconds. Strain! Raise *the shoulders only*, not your back or neck. Now, reverse the process. Press your shoulders as far back as they will go. And hold! You may find that you are lifting your upper torso slightly off the bed. Good! A five full second count, then release.

Now tense the chest muscles. Do this by pressing the palms of your hands against your hips or thighs. Press hard! Count to five — and release.

The arms

Clench your fists and tighten every muscle in your forearms, upper arms and shoulders. Strain! Your entire arms must be rigid. Hold for a slow five, and relax.

Now, open your fists and stretch your fingers and thumbs as widely as possible — fingertips turned down as though you are trying to pick up a basketball from above. Strain! Hold for five, and release.

The lower body

Pause for a moment before going on to your lower body. Take one yawn-breath and lie still. If a second follows, good. Let the full weight of your torso bear down on the bed, *every muscle slack*. Let the bed bear your entire weight. You will feel the tension departing your neck and arms and upper body, and it's a good feeling. Thirty seconds to a minute is enough, then back to work.

Knees bent, suck in the stomach muscles and simultaneously tense the buttocks. At the same time, press the small of your back against the bed and elevate the groin area (a modified pelvic tilt; of which more in the next chapter). Hold for a slow five, and release.

Tense the muscles of your thighs and calves. Hard! You may experience cramping in the arches of your feet or the calves of your legs. If so, simply bring up your toes to counter it.

RELAXATION AWARENESS

Let us pause here to review before continuing. The purpose of the exercises described above was to draw taut each of the muscles of your body, maintain it briefly in a stressed state and then release it. The objective was to fatigue the muscle slightly, thus preparing it for relaxation. It is important, therefore, as you conclude the flexing of each area, to remember to let the muscles go completely slack before continuing.

Concentrate on your body's state of relaxation. Visualize every ounce of your weight bearing down on the bed or the chair. Review in a lazy fashion the diminished tension in your body from the head to the shoulders and arms, to the chest and belly, to the legs and feet. Note how heavy each part of your body feels. You may find that you are ready to fall asleep. If the time and place is appropriate, go ahead.

A final word: you may choose to do each exercise twice before moving to the next and may find it useful to increase the count during each routine from five to ten. Suit yourself. Know this, however: if, when you have completed the sequence and are lying relaxed, you do not *feel* your muscles to be pleasantly slack, you didn't work hard enough at it.

Do these relaxation exercises any time you feel unduly tense. They are particularly effective last thing at night, as they will also help you to fall sleep naturally.

RELAXING YOUR MIND

It is pointless to relax the body if you cannot quiet the mind. Exercise may draw the tension from your muscles, but if, when it is completed, you go back to fretting about your problems, the benefits will soon dissipate and you will be back where you began.

Tension begins in the brain. It may manifest itself in the muscles but it has its origin in the mind.

The mind's off-switch

A problem many face is an inability to turn off the mind when — like an automobile engine with the accelerator stuck — it is running at full speed, out of control. A restless, runaway mind is its most destructive when you are trying to relax.

Here are two suggestions that may help you turn the Off-switch. Begin by examining briefly the problem that is dominating your thoughts. Recognize that there is little you can do about the problem at the moment and resolve to take specific action in the morning.

Now, give your worry a name. It may be the name of a person, an organization, an obligation, anything. *Whatever it is, give it a one-word name.*

Now, close your eyes, take an imaginary piece of chalk and print the name large on a blackboard. Do it with slow deliberation and observe yourself doing it. Make each letter of the word clearly legible. The name completed, place a period at the end of it. The period is important.

Now, take an imaginary eraser and slowly wipe the name off the board. Watch yourself doing it.

Concentrate on doing it deliberately, one letter at a time, erasing each letter entirely, watching it disappear. When the name is gone, erase the period, and as you do, speak the word, "Erase!" It's not a bad idea to say it out loud.

What are you doing? You are banishing the problem by wiping it from your mind. You are not neglecting it or evading it; you are putting it out of your thoughts until the time is appropriate to deal with it.

If the word returns, take the eraser and obliterate it again, letter by letter. Erase the period this time with even greater firmness. Say it: "*Erase!*" Any time it returns, wipe it out and tell it to be gone.

Concentrate. You will be surprised at how completely you can banish disturbing thoughts.

Crowding out your problems

An excellent means for getting rid of tension-inducing thoughts is simply to crowd them out of your mind. Leave them no room into which to intrude.

Here's how.

Delegate to your mind a simple, meaningless assignment. But take note: *it must be one that moves in a sequence and takes a minimal amount of thought.*

Let us suggest the following pattern.

Assign to your mind the following sequence of numbers, making the calculations only in your mind, and in a slow, lazy cadence, *not* speaking them aloud: "*One and* one is two . . . *Two* and one is three . . . *Three* and one is four . . . *Four* and one is five . . . *Five* and one is six," and so on.

Or try counting backwards from a hundred to zero.

The point of the exercise is this: *it keeps your brain occupied while requiring only the most minimal application of your mind.* The objective is simply to bar other thoughts from intruding. Your pet worry may try to sneak in, but your mind will signal, "Sorry. I'm busy."

It is, of course, possible to think of two things at once and you may find yourself doing this. If so, assign to your brain a calculation that demands slightly more concentration. Example: a pattern based on the alphabet: A–A . . . A–B . . . B–B . . . B–C . . . C–C . . . C–D . . . D–D . . . D–E, and so on.

Need something requiring a little more concentration? Go through the alphabet, attaching a man's name to each letter: "A-Al . . . B-Bernie . . . C- Carl . . . D-Don . . . E-Edward," etc. If you haven't fallen asleep by Zeke, do it again with women's names.

Or make up your own pattern.

It doesn't matter what the pattern is as long as it requires little concentration and can be sounded silently in the mind in a slow, measured cadence.

You are guarding your mind against intrusion by thoughts that trouble you and create tension, and you are doing this by occupying your mind with a task that takes the smallest possible amount of concentration. The exercise may seem childish but it works. Try it.

First thing you know, you will be asleep.

19

A Minimal Exercise Program

IF YOU ARE SUBJECT TO RECURRING BACK PROB-
lems, this is the most important chapter in this book.

The facts are clear and are borne out in all the research
done on back pain, its nature and its causes. They are
these:

- Having suffered a serious back problem, you are four
  times as likely to have a second one.
- Each subsequent attack is likely to be more severe
  than those that preceded it.
- The way to avoid future back problems is by keeping
  your back fit through a program of exercise and by so
  training your subconscious mind that you will automatically avoid those actions that might put you in
  jeopardy.

There can be little doubt but that most victims of back
pain plan to begin a program of exercises as soon as they
are up and about again. Nor can there be much doubt
that, having followed the program for a few days or a few
weeks, they will drop it.

It is normal human behavior. We all make resolutions and break them. The first days or weeks in January bear witness to a tendency we all have: to make promises to ourselves that we don't keep.

- We vow to lose weight, and then find that slice of chocolate cake irresistible.
- We vow to quit smoking and then, in a moment of tension, light up.
- We vow to live within a budget and then can't resist that very special purchase.
- We vow to clean out the garage or the attic but can't seem to find the time.
- We vow to dedicate more time to our children but don't.

It is so easy to take the easy road, to postpone the unpleasant, to indulge ourselves. All of us have at some time accepted Oscar Wilde's dictum: "The only way to get rid of a temptation is to yield to it."

VALID EXCUSES

There are persuasive reasons for exercising. There are equally persuasive reasons for not exercising:

- I'm afraid I'll injure myself and put myself back in bed.
- It's hard work.
- I don't have time in the morning.
- I'm too tired at night.
- There's no use starting; I *know* I won't go through with it.
- I'm not sure it will make any real difference.
- My back is back to normal and all I have to do now is be careful.

It is a common failing: you postpone doing your work-out one day for valid reasons and then find it easy to postpone it on day two — and still easier on subsequent days.

The question then becomes: all this being so, is there any point in reading this chapter?

Rather than our listing "Ten Good Reasons Why You Should Undertake a Regimen of Exercise for Your Back," put to yourself the following questions, pausing at the end of each question to reread it:

- Realizing that an unfit back is an acute attack waiting to happen, are you prepared to live with the realization that, *at any careless moment*, you may make the mistake that will temporarily incapacitate you?
- Are you willing to accept the pain you endured last time, knowing that next time it is likely to be worse and to last longer?
- Are you prepared to undergo again those days of incarceration in bed, with the discomfort, the inconvenience and the dislocation of your own and others' lives?
- Realizing that you may incur loss of income and perhaps medical costs if you are sidelined, are you prepared to take those losses?
- Realizing that you may be seriously limited for a period of time in your role as homemaker, are you prepared to endure the anxiety and the practical problems that this will bring to your family?

The responses to each question are so obvious that the point needs no elaboration. The only question is: will you be stimulated to action?

MUSCLE WEAKNESS
The fundamental misconception among laymen is that back trouble has to do with the spine.

Yes, there are back problems caused by disease, by structural malformation and by serious accident, but they are in the minority. Most back pain has nothing to do with the spine as such; it has to do with the muscles and the nervous system that support and activate the spine. And, like all muscles, those related to the spine must be in reasonably good shape or they will not be able to respond to stimuli from the nervous system and will give way when overstressed.

Would you find it odd if, having been a couch-potato for the past year, your legs weren't up to a three-mile jog through the park? Would it surprise you if, having lifted nothing heavier than a forkful of food in recent months, you were easily bested in an arm-wrestling match? Yet, having done little to exercise the muscles of the back and stomach for months, we are taken by surprise when we suffer a jab of pain after raking the yard or find ourselves immobilized as we bend over to lift a spare tire out of the car trunk.

Use it or lose it! It is a fundamental law of life: neglect to exercise a muscle and it atrophies. Fail to keep your back fit and the muscles will grow flaccid and weak and will, at some unexpected and inopportune time, betray you.

So, face the fact: *fail to keep your back in shape and you are going to have problems.*

THREE LEVELS OF EXERCISE

One of the factors that keeps many from beginning a regimen of daily exercise is the tendency to think in ultimates. When it comes to exercise, we tell ourselves that it is pointless to begin unless we are willing to go for broke. And because this is a forbidding prospect, we do nothing.

And little wonder. You pick up most books on back problems and there are pages and pages of exercises — more often than not, more than are needed. Your imagination envisions the sweaty effort, the daily drudgery and the sometime pain involved, and your high resolves go out the window.

But there is no need to become a back-fitness buff. Better to do the necessary minimum than to do nothing at all. So, to encourage those who may tend to do nothing because they are not prepared to do everything, let us make it as simple and easy as possible.

Fact One: *You don't need to exercise every day.* Four days a week will get and keep your back reasonably fit. You may not progress as rapidly as the person who diligently works out every day but you can reach and maintain a satisfactory level of back fitness by exercising, say, Tuesdays, Thursdays and weekends.

Fact Two: *You don't need to start with a complicated series of exercises.* You can begin with three (each of them basic, none of them very difficult) and add others, one by one, as the days go by. What's more, even the complete routine won't require more than ten minutes a day.

Fact Three: *The rewards of back exercise come quickly.* After a week or so, you will be so encouraged by the results — with the sense of accomplishment and the increasing confidence you feel in your back — that your general outlook on life will improve.

The bottom line is this: the program outlined in this chapter does not try to make an athlete out of you, or a fitness buff. Its goal is to bring you to an acceptable level of back-fitness.

Discussing muscular fitness is pointless unless the basic question is asked: fitness for *what*? Watch a competitive gymnast, a downhill skier, a professional football player, an Olympic wrestler on television — you don't *need* that level of fitness. If you are young or particularly vigorous and want to achieve it and are willing to pursue it, fine, but what we are discussing here is an operating level of fitness — *getting your back in shape so that you can do what you have to do or want to do without pain or strain.*

THE MINIMAL BACK-EXERCISE PROGRAM

We present in the following pages two levels of exercise: one for the individual who wants to do as little as possible but as much as necessary; and a second level for those who want to go beyond that and commit the time and effort required to achieve exceptional back fitness.

Before you begin, recognize the obvious: exercise of any kind requires stressing muscles. You are presumably coming off or have a history of some kind of back pain. Most back problems are simple and uncomplicated, but a minority are not. If, when you begin, there is an increase in your pain — a significant increase, not slight discomfort or an occasional twinge — stop and check with your doctor.

In any case, don't begin if you are still suffering acute pain or frequent muscle spasm; you may experience a setback or do yourself injury. On the other hand, don't excuse yourself because there is some general soreness or weakness in the area. Take it easy to begin with and that will soon pass.

Be aware as you begin that there is some truth in the saying, "No pain, no gain." When was the last time you got something worthwhile for nothing?

Getting started

Understand as you begin what your immediate goals are. They are to strengthen your back and stomach muscles and other related areas so that you won't, as the saying has it, "put your back out" again.

"Hold on a minute," you may say: "I understand that the back muscles need to be fit, but why the stomach muscles?" Simply because, in many physical activities (bending, lifting, reaching, twisting, etc.) the back and the stomach muscles work in tandem, each making the other's job easier, each reducing the strain on the other. And if you realize this, you will understand why we begin as we do and why we progress as we do.

Here's an advance look at what's ahead:

- We'll begin with three simple but fundamental exercises.
- We will do them once a day for the first week, and do only five repetitions. Do them twice a week from Week Two.
- Each session will take, at most, five to seven minutes. Two of the exercises are easy; one is a bit harder. You will be pleasantly surprised at how little discomfort they induce and will become aware of a significant increase in your confidence as each day goes by.
- Beginning with Week Two, we will add three more exercises and will stay with these six for the remainder of the month.
- Beginning with Month Two, we will increase the number of repetitions — and that's it.
- Each session will take less than ten minutes.
- After Month Two you can, if you wish, cut the sessions from two a day to one.

As we begin, let it be clear that the exercises detailed below and the number of repetitions suggested are designed for the neophyte, the individual who has never done back exercises or is in the early stages of recovery from a back attack. Those who have previously undertaken an exercise program and neglected it, should follow the routines outlined below but should, at least, double the number of repetitions. You are the best judge.

WEEK ONE

1. The pelvic tilt

The pelvic tilt is basic to many back exercises. It is particularly useful in stretching the muscles of the lower back and in strengthening the stomach. As well, it eases the pressure on the facet joints. Beyond that, it is the starting position for most of the exercises in which you bend forward, the so-called flexion exercises.

Its primary value is, however, preventive. By using it as you exercise, you minimize the risk of injury. Beyond that, the pelvic tilt helps to produce better posture, which will, in itself, help prevent back problems.

A word of encouragement as you begin Exercise One: because back pain can be so frightening, many approach even the simplest exercise with trepidation. In this case, don't — you can't hurt yourself learning the pelvic tilt, so relax.

Don't be discouraged if you have some difficulty following the directions given. The pelvic tilt is among the simplest of exercises but it is difficult to explain. Persevered in, it will soon become as natural as breathing.

We suggest that you begin on the bed rather than on the floor for the simple reason that it is easier for a person who has not yet fully recovered from a back attack to lie on a bed than to get down to and up from the floor. However, if your bed sags, put a blanket on the floor.

Here's how it's done:

1. Lie on your back, arms by your sides, legs moderately bent, your feet flat on the bed or floor (see Figure 1). Use a pillow if you wish, but not a thick one.

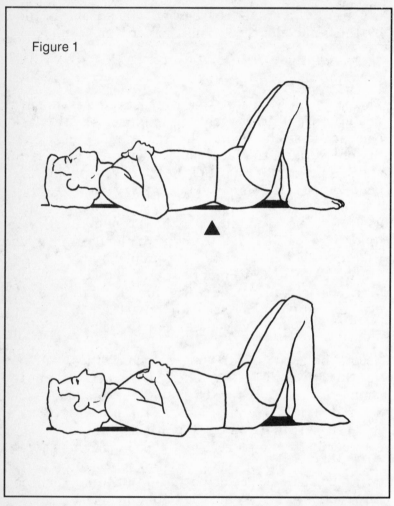

Figure 1

2. Tighten your stomach muscles and tilt your pelvis so that the pubic area is raised. Don't raise your hips off the bed and don't put any extra weight on your feet. What you are doing is reversing the normal arch of your back, making it bow outward, and, in doing so, stretching the muscles involved.

3. Repeat the action a total of five times for starters. Hold each time for a slow count of five. Don't hold your breath; breathe normally.

It may give you a better sense of what you are trying to accomplish if, before you begin, you place a hand beneath your back. You will feel a space where the arch is. Press the small of your back against you hand. That's the desired movement.

Once you've learned the pelvic tilt, *use it to begin every exercise session*.

Later, you should learn to do the pelvic tilt while standing. It's a bit more difficult but you will master it after a try or two. Stand with your back to a wall, your shoulders and buttocks touching it, your feet close but not necessarily touching it. Now, tilt your pelvis, just as you do when lying down, and maintain it in that position. Now assume the position away from the wall. It's not easy but neither is it all that difficult. The point is: it is useful in a number of ways. If you have been standing for an extended time, assume the pelvic tilt for a few minutes. It eases the pressures on your low back, stretches the muscles and helps relax them.

2. The low-back stretch
This is an invaluable exercise. It will stretch and strengthen your low-back muscles, separate the joints in the spine and help tone the hamstring muscles in the back of the thighs. As well, it will ease the soreness in the low-back area and is particularly useful if you have strained a facet joint or are suffering from inflammation as a result of having done so.

1. Begin by assuming and maintaining the pelvic tilt.
2. Raise your knees toward your chest — one leg at a time if you are a beginner.

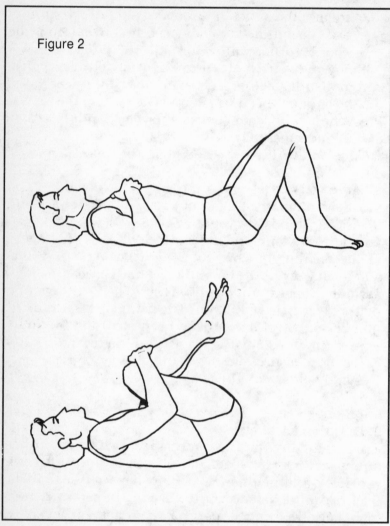

Figure 2

3. Grasp your legs at the knees and, slowly but firmly, pull your thighs toward your chest. (See Figure 2.) Begin gently. Increase the pressure until there is the beginning of discomfort. Ease off slightly and

maintain that position for a slow count of five. If you are overweight you may find your stomach in the way. If so, spread your thighs.

4. Release and lower your legs *slowly*. If you prefer, lower one leg at a time.
5. Repeat for a total of five times.

(If your problem is a disc protrusion, this exercise could lead to an increase in pain. If that happens, stop, and if you haven't done so, check it out.)

3. The semi situp

The semi situp is an isotonic exercise, meaning simply that it contracts the stomach muscles. The muscles, fully tensed, do not move.

The primary objective here is to strengthen your stomach muscles. If yours are out of shape, this exercise will be somewhat demanding. But don't duck it; strong stomach muscles are fundamental to a fit back. If your back is still painful from the initial attack, postpone until after the pain has eased.

1. Lie on your back and assume the pelvic tilt.
2. Raise your head, tucking your chin close to your neck. (See Figure 3.)
3. Arms straight, raise your neck and shoulders off the bed and reach out until your hands are beside your knees. Do *not* try to sit up, and remember to maintain the pelvic tilt.
4. Hold it briefly the first time you try it. After that, hold for a count of five. It's a bit difficult to breathe normally but you will manage it after a while. When you release, *don't fall back*; slowly lower, first your shoulders, then your head.
5. Repeat for a total of five times.

Continue these three exercises daily for the first week.

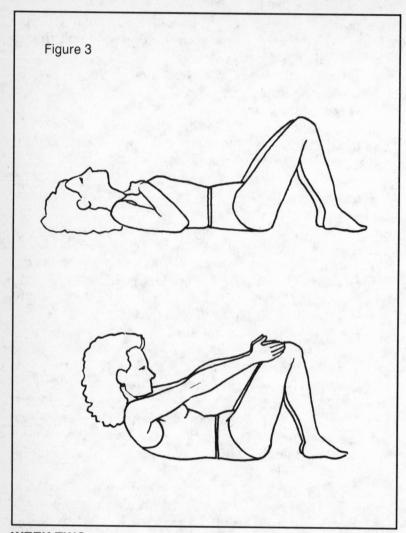

Figure 3

WEEK TWO

4. Pulling strings
Time now to add three additional exercises. The three
flexion exercises you have been doing are designed primarily to stretch the muscles of your back while, at the

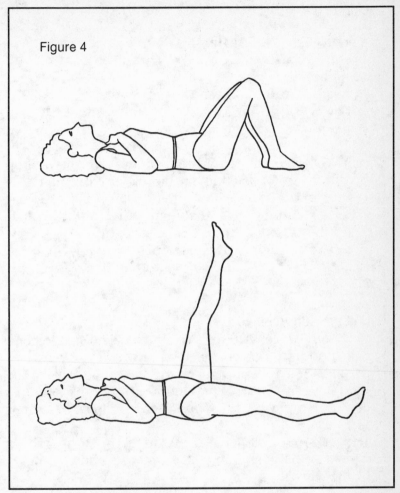

Figure 4

same time, strengthening your stomach muscles. But there is another set of muscles that plays an important part in supporting and assisting the back — the hamstrings.

The hamstrings are the muscles that run from the pelvis down the back of the thigh to the knee, and it is not uncommon for them to tighten in response to chronic pain. This relative inflexibility then restricts the mobility of the spine, which, in combination, will tend to make you bend and lift in the wrong way.

1. Lie on your back, arms by your sides or at rest on your chest.
2. Assume and maintain the pelvic tilt.
3. Lower your right leg until it is flat against the bed.
4. Keeping it straight, raise the right leg (See Figure 4.) and slowly bring it as close to vertical as you can. (It is not necessary to bring it to a full vertical.) Stop when you feel strong discomfort or extreme tightness in the back of your thigh or lower back. Hold it for a count of five and *slowly* return it to the floor, taking care to keep the knee straight.
5. Rest for a moment, consciously relaxing the muscle. Repeat the exercise for a total of five repetitions.
6. Do the same with your left leg.

5. The push-me/pull-you

In addition to strengthening the muscles needed to bend forward and straighten up, it is important to work on those muscles that enable you to rotate the trunk of the body. They are crucial in playing such sports as tennis or golf, and in everyday life when there is a need to turn or twist.

The push-me/pull-you is useful in further toning those all-important stomach muscles and, as a bonus, it helps trim the waistline.

The exercise consists of simply pushing with an opposing hand against your raised knee and is easily controlled in terms of the amount of effort expended.

1. Lie on your back and assume the pelvic tilt.
2. Raise your left leg, keeping it bent, to the point where your thigh is vertical.

Figure 5

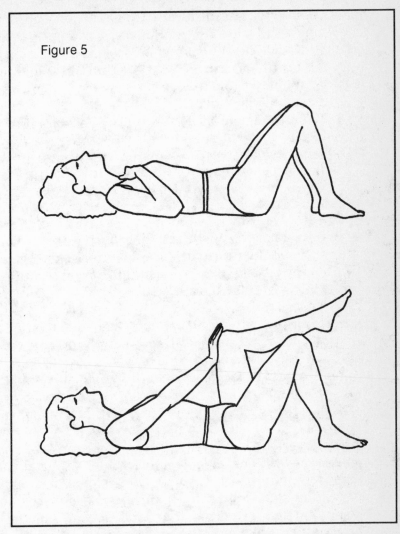

3. Maintaining the pelvic tilt, place the palm of your *right* hand against your *left* knee. (See Figure 5.)You may find it more comfortable to raise your head and shoulders, tucking in your chin.

4. Keeping your arm straight, push firmly against the knee while resisting sufficiently with the leg to keep it motionless. If you feel pain, ease off a touch but maintain pressure. Sustain that pressure for a count of five and then, slowly, lower the leg and the head and shoulders.

5. Rest a moment and then repeat, for a total of five repetitions, with the same leg. Switch legs and arms for the same number of repetitions. Begin with fewer if you wish.

6. The sloppy pushup

Everyone has done pushups. Their purpose was to build arm and shoulder muscles, and few things do it better. The sloppy pushup differs inasmuch as you *do not* keep your back straight, and your purpose is entirely different.

On your first attempt, particularly if you are still feeling pain from your back attack, simply lie face down. Difficult as it may be to believe, you are now doing an extension exercise. The face-down, prone position arches your back and helps strengthen the paraspinal muscles, the two heavy-duty muscles that run alongside your spine.

Turning your head, place a hand or a forearm under your face — whichever feels comfortable. Now, stay there for a few minutes. If lying on your stomach produces pain, and especially if the pain increases or seems to spread farther away from the spine, discontinue the exercise and check it out. (If there is any significant sag in your mattress, do this exercise on the floor.)

On Day Two, prop yourself up on your elbows, putting yourself in the position so popular with children when they lie on the floor to watch television. Remain so for a slow count of five. Repeat as many as five times unless it becomes uncomfortable.

On Day Three, place your hands beside your shoulders, just as you would in preparing to do a standard pushup. Now, raise your torso to the full length of your arms but *don't raise your hips or legs*. Let your back sag. Count five and then lower your trunk. Use your arm muscles only.

Five repetitions at each stage if you're up to it. Otherwise, work up to that number over the next fews days.

An Extra: Doin' the Squat

Fundamental to avoiding back strain is proper lifting. Whenever possible, any heavy lifting should be done with the legs, not the back.

But if you are going to assign the responsibility to the legs (mostly the thigh muscles), it is essential to build their strength. And the easiest way to do this is to practice squatting.

It's a simple-enough matter:

1. Put a hand on a chair or any object that will provide a stable point of balance.
2. Keeping your back straight, simply bend your knees halfway — to where the thighs are more or less horizontal. (See Figure 6.) It is *not* necessary to go all the way down; as a matter of fact, it is hard on the knee joints, so don't.
3. Hold for a count of five and straighten up. Repeat to a total of five.

If you are out of shape, you may be surprised to find that you can do only three squats the first time you try. But you will make swift progress and will soon be able to do a dozen or more repetitions without undue effort.

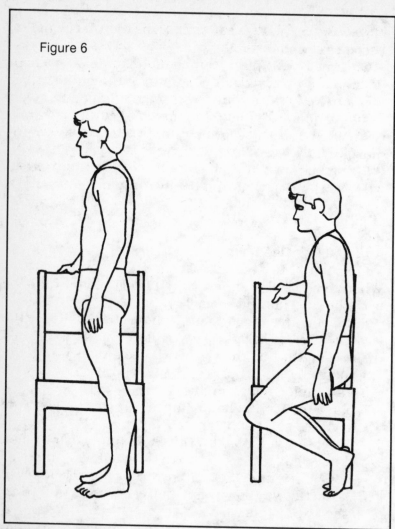

Figure 6

A FINAL WORD

The seven exercises described above are all you need to reach an acceptable degree of back fitness. They are basic. If, however, yours is an active life or if your job calls for manual labor, you will want to go beyond them, and you should. You will find a variety of back-exercise books available in the library and in bookstores to give you guidance in working out your own program.

One final point needs emphasizing: *neglect the minimal exercises outlined in these pages (or others comparable to them) and you are almost certainly going to suffer further back problems.* Fail to maintain a reasonable degree of back fitness and the occasional back pain you experience can become chronic. Exercise, and these occasional problems will, in all likelihood, disappear.

Beyond all else remember this: your back attack was a warning — heed it!

The Automatic Response System

A Foolproof Way to End Back Attacks

ALL THAT PRECEDES THIS CHAPTER IS PROLOGUE. We have learned something of the causes of back pain, how to deal with an acute attack, how to manage the trauma and how to live in the knowledge that one is never entirely free of the possibility of a recurrence of the problem.

But the promise in the title of this book is that there is a foolproof way to end back attacks. May the reader hold a reasonable expectation that this promise can be kept?

The answer is an unequivocal yes!

DIFFERENT REACTIONS

There appear to be two general patterns in the responses of individuals to an attack of acute back pain.

The majority of sufferers treat the attack with bed rest, analgesics and a variety of other means. The acute phase soon passes. In nine of ten cases (regardless of the treatment given, or not given), the symptoms disappear in a few days or a few weeks and the patient returns to normal. Usually, a regimen of exercises is begun but is soon abandoned. Other attacks follow.

The minority of sufferers treat the initial attack in more or less the same way and enter into a similar regimen of exercise. These people, however, persevere in their quest for back fitness, and while they may suffer an occasional relapse, the problem does not normally become chronic.

Are we suggesting with this comparison that most back trouble can be ended by following a set of specialized exercises? Of course not. As important as exercise is to the maintenance of a healthy back — and it is fundamental — it offers no guarantee against future back attacks. You may, in a moment of carelessness, or recklessness, or indifference, put yourself in a place of jeopardy.

How then may one hope to escape the recurring cycle of trauma-and-recovery, to go beyond fitness and vigilance? We propose in this chapter to put forward a solution that will enable you to banish the specter of recurring back attacks through *the creation of an Automatic Response System in your subconscious mind.*

BACK ATTACKS ARE PREDICTABLE

A severe back attack seldom comes without warning. We may have failed to recognize it or heed it but the warning was there. The reason for the onset can usually be identified by the doctor, the patient or both. Unfortunately, it is usually with the wisdom of hindsight.

As we have seen, a variety of circumstances tend to precipitate most back attacks. The most common are:
- You have let yourself get out of shape.
- You have overdone some physical activity.
- You have come through a period of heightened tension.

- The tension has been intensified by fatigue.
- You are having problems at work.
- You are facing financial difficulties.
- You are experiencing conflicts in a relationship.
- Your family life is stressful.
- You are in the mid-term or late months of a pregnancy.

Most of us, at various times in our lives, find ourselves facing one or more of the situations listed above, and there is no avoiding some of them. The question then arises: if these are the primary causes of back attacks and are an inevitable part of contemporary life, what can one do to avoid recurring back trouble?

The answer is: *to train your subconscious mind to recognize the circumstances that precede a seizure and automatically to take the necessary steps to avoid it.*

Can the subconscious mind be so conditioned? The answer is an unequivocal yes. As a matter of fact, most of the things we learn in life and most of the habits we form are the result of such a process. The process is called *building conditioned reflexes*.

TRAINING THE SUBCONSCIOUS

We come into life as helpless, uncoordinated infants, and the various skills we acquire are the result of learning to control our reflexes.

What is a newborn child? It is an utterly dependent human being with virtually no control over itself or its environment. It can't focus its eyes. It can't coordinate its legs and arms. It has no sense of balance. It can't control its bowel and kidney functions, even the swallowing of its saliva.

Yes, it has inherited a few survival reflexes: it will suck when put to the breast, it will flinch if in danger of falling and it will grasp a finger placed within its hand. But, to survive, it will have to learn virtually everything else: to turn over, to lift its head, to sit up, to get onto its hands and knees, to feed itself, to control its body functions, to walk . . .

How are such life skills acquired? By learning, through trial and error, to control our muscular processes. That is the way we learn to walk, to run, to skate, to throw a ball, to dance, to knit, to drive a car, to play a piano, to operate a computer, to fly an airplane.

These and the thousands of other things we do in everyday life are made possible as the result of lodging information in the subconscious. And they are based on conditioning our reflexes.

THE CONTROL OF YOUR BODY

First, understand that everything that happens in your body is controlled by one of three nervous systems: the central nervous system, the autonomic nervous system and the involuntary reflex system.

The central nervous system is controlled by the brain and directs the volitional actions of the body. Through the central nervous system, the brain "orders" the muscles to function as required to achieve its objectives.

The autonomic nervous system governs what might be described as the vital functions: heartbeat, blood pressure, breathing, constriction or enlargement of the iris of the eye, etc. You have virtually no control over them.

By way of illustration: try to stop breathing. You can will yourself to hold your breath for an extended period of time but, within a minute or two at most, you will learn that, try as you may, your autonomic nervous system will not permit it.

Nor can you control actions governed by *the involuntary reflex system*. They are activated by nerve impulses that bypass the brain.

Example: If you tap the tendon below the kneecap, the stimulus doesn't move to the brain; it takes a short cut, traveling to the spinal cord and directly back to the muscle of the leg. The reflex is involuntary. You may try to control the jerk of your leg, but you can't.

There are, however, some involuntary reflexes that you *can* learn to control, and these are the key to avoiding back attacks. Such learned responses are called *conditioned reflex actions*.

CONDITIONING YOUR REFLEXES

Most of our reflex actions are inherited. They are essentially survival mechanisms.

Aeons ago, the body learned to protect itself by reacting, without conscious thought, to danger. You observe this reflex operating when you shudder and jerk away from a stimulus such as, say, a spider crawling on your skin. You don't choose to so react; your body draws back automatically in an attempt to avoid potential pain.

The reaction is involuntary.

The important point is: *you can learn to control such involuntary reactions*.

Example: When a nurse brings a hypodermic needle to your arm your body tends to flinch, to draw away. But your brain overrules the normal reflex, and you submit to the needle.

Such a "learned" response is known as *a conditioned reflex*. The subconscious has learned to disregard its normal response and to react to a particular set of circumstances in another way.

This is the key to protecting yourself from a sudden back attack: *train your subconscious to recognize those* circumstances that might overstress the muscles of the back and to take protective action.

Nor is this difficult to do; we do similar things every day.

CONDITIONING THE MIND TO AVOID TROUBLE

From birth we have lodged in the subconscious mind thousands of responses to potentially dangerous situations, defensive actions taken automatically when danger is sensed.

For example:

- At the ballpark, you don't have to *think* about ducking when a foul-tip ricochets off the hitter's bat toward your head — it is a conditioned reflex.
- When a child darts into her path, the driver of a car hits the brakes without thinking — it is an automatic reaction, a conditioned reflex.
- A mother, her attention focused on a multitude of household duties, reacts to the slightest extraordinary sound from the upstairs nursery — it is a conditioned reflex

The reasons these individuals react as they do is obvious: *each has conditioned the subconscious mind to recognize a particular set of circumstances and to react automatically in an appropriate way.*

Our days are filled with actions taken without conscious thought. When, as a child in first grade, you were presented with a new word, you had to learn to recognize each individual letter, then the order in which they were arranged and, finally, to imprint on your memory the meaning of the word. Now, your eyes scan a printed page and, without pausing to "think," you get the meaning.

You have trained your subconscious to react.

As a stenographer types a letter, does she have to think about the positions of the individual characters on the keyboard? She once had to; but no more. She has so conditioned her subconscious that, without her consciously commanding it to, it activates the responses in her fingers.

Using this process, you must train your subconscious to monitor the movements of and the messages from your body and to initiate, *automatically*, the actions required to protect you from a move that might overstress the muscles of your back.

How can you do this?

By establishing in your subconscious mind a set of automatic responses to the demands being made on your body, demands that, in a particular situation, might strain the muscles of your back.

You must make these responses as much "second nature" as glancing to the left when you step off the curb into the street. Forget to look to the left and you may end up in hospital or at the morgue. The point is: you *don't* forget — your subconscious protects you from potential injury.

Indeed, some automatic responses become so firmly fixed in the mind that it can be exceedingly difficult to "unlearn" them. If you have visited the British Isles, where the traffic travels in the left lane, you have probably had the experience of endangering yourself when, stepping from the curb, you looked the "wrong" way.

We have all had the experience of walking down an escalator that has been taken out of operation. Your mindset about an escalator's movement is so ingrained that it is almost impossible to descend the steps normally. In a reverse situation: ride a moving sidewalk of the type found at airports and, no matter how you may prepare yourself to step off in stride at the end, you almost invariably stumble.

These are precisely the type of conditioned reflexes needed to protect your back.

You may object: "Hold on a moment! If I follow this advice I'll become obsessed with guarding my back and become a kind of cripple; constantly limiting my physical activity and letting the memory of a past problem dominate the remainder of my life. And I will progressively weaken my back muscles by forever babying them."

Not so.

As your back muscles move to full recovery, you will discover that your brain has a mind of its own. Your subconscious mind will adapt to the fact that there are fewer pain signals coming from a specific area and will increasingly return healthy, normal responses.

Beyond that, if you follow the counsel in the preceding chapter, you will strengthen the relevant muscles through the regimen of exercises described there.

THE BODY'S ADAPTABILITY

Some years ago a friend almost severed the thumb of his left hand while doing some carpentry. The power handsaw, bound in a compressed cut, leaped backward when started up, severing the bone at the lower knuckle and leaving the thumb hanging by a ragged piece of tissue. A surgeon specializing in the human hand repaired it brilliantly, although the thumb is now shorter than the right one and can't quite be straightened out.

As it healed, and for weeks afterwards, the victim avoided using the thumb. Then, progressively, as the pain eased and the accident retreated to the back of his consciousness, completely forgot about the injury and now use both hands equally, favoring neither.

So, don't worry about indulging your back during the recovery period. Granted, to continue to do so after it has returned to normal would cause the muscles to atrophy and would, indeed, turn you into a semi-invalid. But once the injury has passed and you have strengthened the affected muscles and gone on to train your subconscious to recognize potentially risky circumstances, there is no reason why you should suffer that kind of injury again.

AN EARLY-RESPONSE SYSTEM

Think of the procedure as an "Automatic Response System." You program your subconscious to recognize the circumstances that could bring about an overstressing of the muscles of the back and to counter that jeopardy *automatically*.

Here is a simple example of how it works.

A sufferer from chronic back pain was at lunch with a friend. The conversation was prolonged. The restaurant was noisy, and for the better part of an hour and a half he found himself required to lean forward — a fatiguing posture — to eat and to hear what was being said.

As he rose to leave, his friend said, "Still having trouble with your back, I see?"

"No," he said. "Not recently. Why?"

"The way you rose from your chair."

The man couldn't remember doing it, but realized immediately what he must have done: he had put his hands on the arms of the chair, slid his buttocks to the edge of the seat, placed his feet beneath his upper body and risen straight up. The entire sequence had been automatic.

To state it more exactly: the conditioned reflexes lodged in his subconscious had recognized the potential for danger in his prolonged, unsupported bending forward and had initiated a sequence of movements designed to avoid overstressing the fatigued muscles of his back.

The actions required to rise from his chair had been taken without his realizing he had made them.

This is the secret for avoiding back seizures: Program your subconscious mind to recognize the circumstances that will put your back at risk, and your conditioned reflexes will act to protect you from injury.

We call it "The Automatic Response System."

How is it established in the mind? By fixing at the forefront of your subconscious the *conditions* and the *circumstances* that could lead to your overstressing the muscles of your back.

DANGEROUS CIRCUMSTANCES

There are easily recognizable circumstances that can put your back at risk. They include:

- *You are out of shape*. Your muscles are slack and weak from lack of exercise.
- *You are fatigued*. You have been making too many demands on your body. Your muscles need rest.
- *You are tense*. Some of your muscles have been drawn taut for a period of hours or days, and lack resiliency.
- *You are stiff*. Your muscles are sore and perhaps swollen from too much physical activity.
- *Your posture is bad*. As a consequence, some of your muscles are fatigued from being under constant stress.
- *You are cold*. Your muscles have contracted as a result of inactivity or being subjected to low temperatures.
- *You are aging*. Some of the strength, endurance and resiliency of your muscles has diminished with the years.

Any of these conditions can lead to a straining of the muscles of the back to the point of injury. If, for instance, you are tense or stiff or cold or out of shape, it is mandatory that, before subjecting your muscles to stress, they be warmed up. If professional athletes find it necessary to do a warmup to protect themselves from injury, how much more imperative it is for the rest of us.

Learn to listen to the language of your body. Become sensitive to the ways in which it communicates. For example: if, after having a nap, you rise and find your muscles stiff, your body will induce a yawn and a desire to stretch. What is it saying? That the inactive muscles need to be invigorated with a fresh supply of oxygen and stretched, having contracted during your rest.

Your Automatic Response system is talking to you.

DANGEROUS ACTIONS

Some of the demands we make on our back muscles are more taxing than others. Some, in certain circumstances, are downright dangerous and can land us in bed. We need to learn what these dangerous actions are, how they lead to injury and how they can be avoided, and then fix them in the subconscious. This is of paramount importance because most back attacks result from a moment of carelessness. When the conscious mind is otherwise engaged, we may act unwisely.

These risky actions include:

- bending over without flexing your knees;
- straightening up quickly after bending over;
- lifting, with the load away from your body;
- turning while lifting;
- prolonged standing;
- sitting with insufficient low-back support;
- rising after lengthy sitting;
- certain sports activities.

Your back is a versatile mechanism but it is vulnerable. Disregard its limitations and you may injure or even incapacitate yourself. This book has one purpose: insofar as it possible (and it *is* possible) to free you from such dangers. But let this be understood from the beginning: no book can of itself guarantee you freedom from back pain or back attacks. That, in the final analysis, is up to you.

ABOUT THE AUTHORS

Charles Templeton

In one extraordinary lifetime, Charles Templeton has achieved recognition in a dozen different fields. He is the author of eleven books, many of which have been sold around the world. One, *The Kidnapping of the President*, has been made into a major motion picture. Other titles include: *Succeeding*, *World of One*, *The Queen's Secret*, *An Anecdotal Memoir*, *The Third Temptation*, *Act of God* and *Jesus: His Life*.

He has been host of numerous television shows in the United States and Canada, and was co-host (with Merv Griffin) of a weekly program on the CBS television network. His daily program, *Dialogue*, with Pierre Berton, was syndicated across Canada for 18 years. In his early years he was one of North America's most successful preachers, speaking to audiences of up to 50,000 at Soldier Field, Chicago, the Rose Bowl, Pasadena, and elsewhere.

Charles Godfrey, MD

Charles Godfrey is one of Canada's most eminent medical practitioners and a world leader in his speciality, physical medicine. He is the director of the department of Rehabilitation Medicine at Wellesley Hospital in Toronto, a Fellow of the Royal College of Physicians and Surgeons (Canada), Professor Emeritus of the Faculty of Medicine, University of Toronto, past president of both the Canadian Association of Physical Medicine.

He has also been a member of the Ontario Provincial Parliament, was the leader of the People or Planes movement and, for his various public services, has been awarded the Order of Canada.

He is the author of *Medicine for Ontario, People or Planes?* and *The Ageless Exercise Plan*.

Index

television, 62–63
tension: apprehension, 158;
  awareness, 161–62;
  "cautionary tension," 96;
  contemporary way of life,
  154–56; fear of recur-
  rence, 66, 70–71; from
  driving, 143–44, 149–51;
  from standing, 130–31;
  hypnotherapy, 21;
  learning to relax, 70–71;
  massage for, 34; proper
  breathing, 163–67;
  relationship between back
  problems and, 12, 156–57;
  relaxation exercises, 167–
  71; relaxing your mind,
  171–73; while seated, 114–
  15
thigh muscles, 70
thoracic vertebrae, 98
toilet, 90–92
torsion flexibility, 148
tranquilizer, 70
Travell, Dr. Janet, 123
trucks, 144
twisting: while lifting or
  bending, 110–12
Tylenol, 28

United States:
  acupuncture, 19;
  Robaxisal, 27

unloading the car, 151–52
upper body: benefits of
  walking, 141; exercise,
  68–69

vertebrae: fracture of, 41–
  42; nature of spine, 39–
  40, 99–100; neck, 111;
  ribs, 98; stress-fractures,
  138
vibrators, 13
visitors, 64–65

walking: benefits of, 135–
  36, 141; frequency, 139;
  jogging or, 136–38;
  monitoring your heart
  rate, 140–41; shoes, 139
warm water, 34, 82
waterbed, 59–61
weight lifters, 109, 129
whirlpool baths, 13
workforce absenteeism,
  155
workplace: office chairs,
  115–20; standing in the,
  132–33

X-rays, 17

yawning, 164–67
yin and yang, 19–20

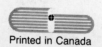

Printed in Canada